DATA PREPARATION AND EXPLORATION

Applied to Healthcare Data

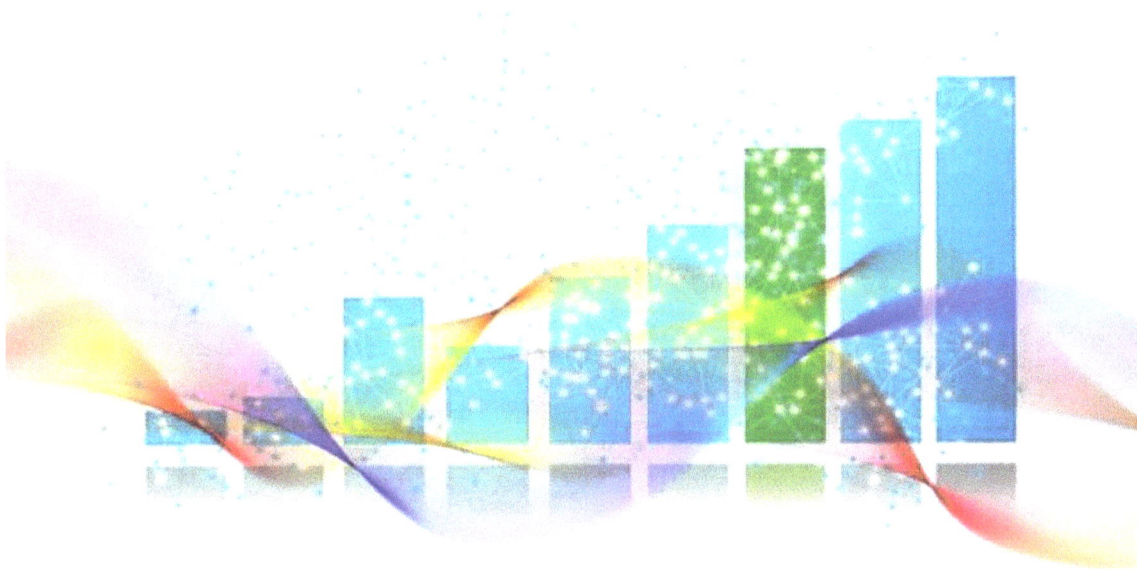

Robert Hoyt MD FACP FAMIA
Associate Clinical Professor, Department of Internal Medicine
Virginia Commonwealth University, Richmond, VA

Robert A. Muenchen MS PSAT
Research Computing Support
University of Tennessee, Knoxville, TN

Data Preparation and Exploration
Applied to Healthcare Data

Disclaimer

Print copy: ISBN: 978-0-9887529-7-9

eBook (pdf): ISBN: 978-0-9887529-0-0

eBook (EPUB): ISBN: 978-0-9887529-6-2

TABLE OF CONTENTS

PREFACE

Most data scientists spend the majority of their time locating appropriate clinical data, then preparing and exploring it for meaningful results. While some have referred to data science as the "sexiest job of the twenty-first century," the reality is that it involves much more than just creating a model with cutting-edge algorithms and programming languages.

Data preparation and exploration is like prep work before painting. There is sanding, dissembling, color selection, and priming before the final coat of paint is applied. Without proper data preparation and exploration, a user will likely encounter a "garbage in, garbage out" scenario.

We wrote this textbook because we felt there was not enough emphasis on this topic and only a few resources to select from. Most resources tend to focus on only one approach, such as applying a programming language to every problem. In this book, we use statistical software, spreadsheets, and programming languages to tackle data preparation and exploration problems. Also, we use healthcare datasets to make the scenarios more real-world and we added student exercises at the end of each chapter. We also added video tutorials in as many places as possible to provide additional resources in another format.

The field is moving towards automated machine learning that will expedite the process of data preparation and exploration. Despite this welcomed advance, budding data scientists will still need to understand why and how these steps are taken.

There is a separate chapter on healthcare data resources to make the journey easier. The datasets are all publicly available and may derive from governmental and private organizations. Instructors and students are strongly urged to "get their feet wet" with as many data exercises as possible. It would be wise to develop a checklist of the normal steps of data preparation and exploration for every dataset you analyze.

More textbook details are available on https://informaticseducation.org

Robert Hoyt MD FACP FAMIA

Robert Muenchen MS PSA

ABOUT THE AUTHORS

Robert E. Hoyt, MD, FACP, FAMIA, is an internal medicine physician who was in private practice for 15 years and served as a physician in the military for 20 years. During this time he taught health informatics for 13 years at the University of West Florida. He has been involved in health informatics for the past two decades, but in the last five years he has focused primarily on biomedical data science, with emphasis on machine learning and artificial intelligence. He is a co-author and co-editor of Health Informatics: Practical Guide that is in its seventh edition. Additionally, he is the co-editor and co-author of the Introduction to Biomedical Data Science with Robert Muenchen that launched in 2019.

Robert A. Muenchen, MS, PSA is the author of the BlueSky Statistics 7.1 User Guide, R for SAS and SPSS Users, and coauthor of R for Stata Users and Introduction to Biomedical Data Science. An ASA Accredited Professional Statistician, Bob wrote or co-authored over 70 articles published in scientific journals and conference proceedings. At The University of Tennessee, he guided more than 1,000 graduate theses and dissertations and he continues to teach R workshops there.

ACKNOWLEDGMENTS

We would like to thank Ann Yoshihashi MD FACE for textbook formatting and proofreading.

We would also like to thank Karen Monsen PhD RN FAMIA FAAN and David Hurwitz MD FACP for their help reviewing the textbook

1

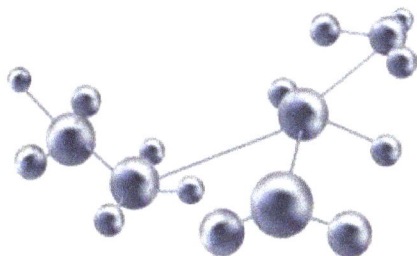

THE IMPORTANCE OF DATA PREPARATION AND EXPLORATION

Robert Hoyt MD   Robert Muenchen

"Data scientists are involved with gathering data, massaging it into a tractable form, making it tell its story, and presenting that story to others." – Mike Loukides, editor, O'Reilly Media.

LEARNING OBJECTIVES

After reading the chapter the reader should be able to:
- Discuss why data must be prepared and explored prior to modeling
- Enumerate the usual steps of data cleaning and exploration
- List the data preparation and exploration methodologies using spreadsheets, statistical packages, and programming languages

INTRODUCTION

Because data scientists and others spend so much time with data preparation and exploration, we believe a separate textbook is warranted and we now offer it in addition to our other textbook Introduction to Biomedical Data Science. (1) Data preparation and exploration occur early in the data science process, as data scientists prepare their data before modeling.

The *data science process,* (as adapted from Blitzstein and Pfeister) includes multiple steps, as displayed in figure 1.1 below. (2) This chapter will focus on the first 4 steps, specifically asking the right question, getting the data, cleaning, visualizing, and exploring the data.

Figure 1.1 The data science process (adapted from Blitzstein and Pfeister)

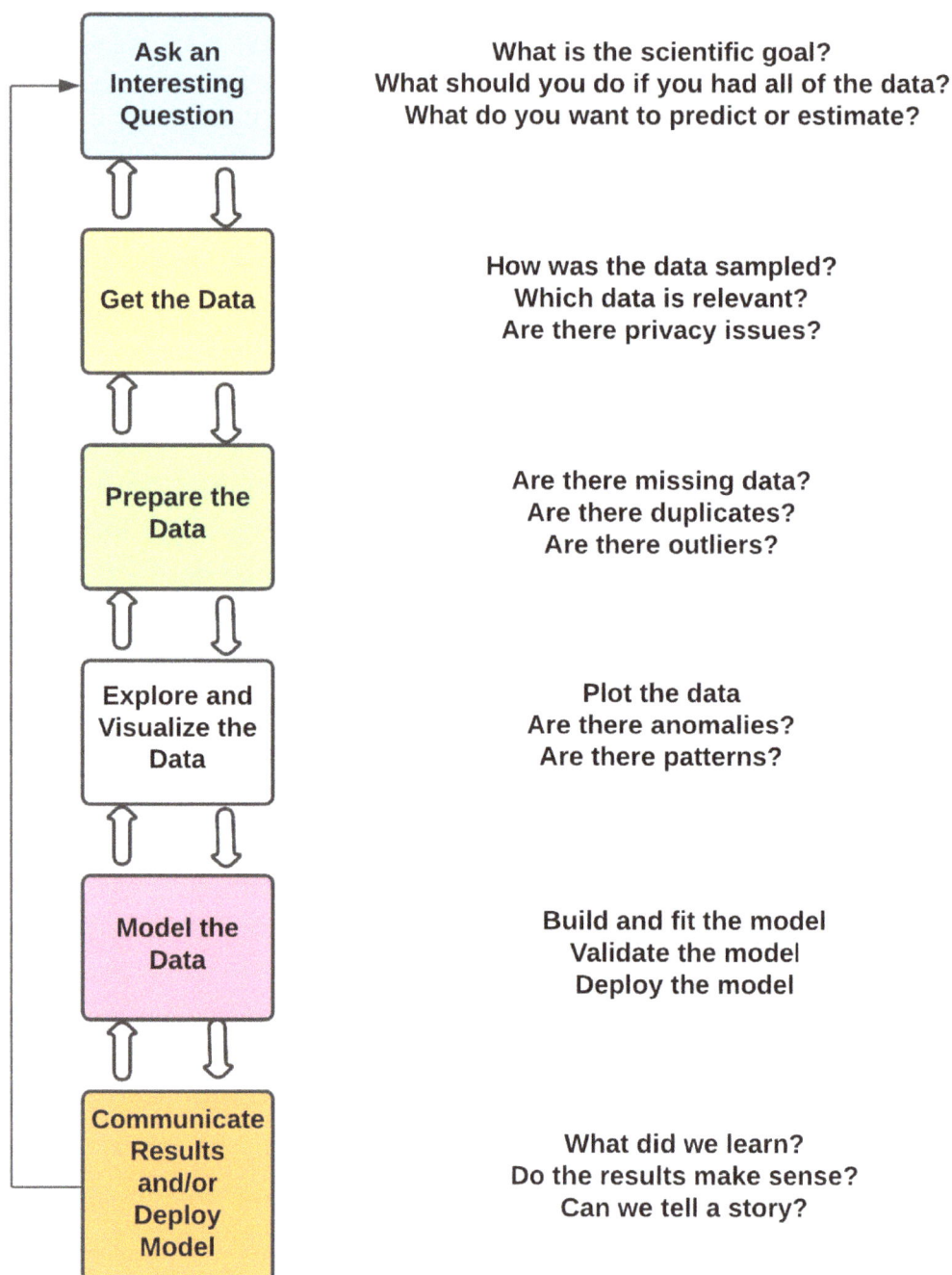

Ask an Interesting Question	**What is the scientific goal?** **What should you do if you had all of the data?** **What do you want to predict or estimate?**
Get the Data	**How was the data sampled?** **Which data is relevant?** **Are there privacy issues?**
Prepare the Data	**Are there missing data?** **Are there duplicates?** **Are there outliers?**
Explore and Visualize the Data	**Plot the data** **Are there anomalies?** **Are there patterns?**
Model the Data	**Build and fit the model** **Validate the model** **Deploy the model**
Communicate Results and/or Deploy Model	**What did we learn?** **Do the results make sense?** **Can we tell a story?**

The majority of the time spent by a data scientist is on the early four steps of the data science process. Take note of the number of bi-directional arrows between the boxes and the single arrow on the left that returns from deploying the model back to the beginning. Starting over happens every time a variable, metric, or feature is added to the dataset. This highlights the possibility that the model created was a poor performer and needs to be adjusted, and the process starts over. This entire process is iterative and not linear. Domain (clinical) expertise is critical to help sort out what is important and what is not.

The overriding focus of a data science project is to fully understand the research question, locate and collect appropriate data, clean and prepare the data, then begin the modeling process. An additional implication is that any member of the data science team can hone their data preparation and exploration skills and that will be a skill as important as running a model or tweaking an algorithm. In addition, every member of the data science team is important and brings a different skill set to the table. VIDEO (3) Figure 1.2 displays a potential healthcare data science team.

Figure 1.2 Healthcare Data Science Team

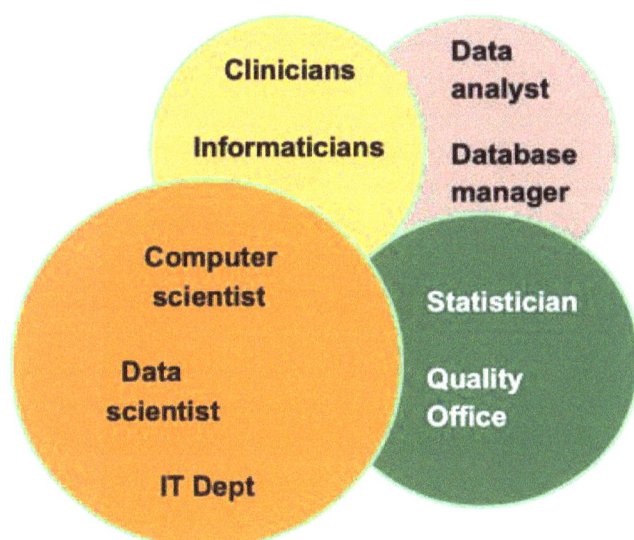

In this chapter, the usual steps to prepare, clean, and explore data prior to the modeling phase will include statistical methods, spreadsheet tools, and programming language methodologies. Of paramount importance is the notion that variables represent clinically-relevant information, and that some depth of understanding about the clinical importance of the question and the variable is requisite to this exploration. There is no universal organization of data preparation and exploration, so what is presented is a common-sense approach. As a reminder, data are plural and datum is singular.

Figure 1.3 tells the story of how the average data scientist spends their time on a data science project. This graph shows that about 19% of their time is spent collecting the data and 60% of the time cleaning and organizing data. Nine percent is spent mining the data; 4 percent refining algorithms; 3 percent training the model and 5 percent doing "other" activities. (4) Keep in mind that this bar chart does not take into account the considerable time spent with the client discussing the problem, presenting/communicating the findings, or deploying the model. It also assumes that the steps of the data science process don't have to be repeated due to problems or errors, which is unrealistic.

Importantly, data science is a team sport. That means that most data science projects occur as a result of a team effort. Every "player" should be considered important and their opinion valued. They may have "corporate knowledge" of 1. How the administration thinks 2. What the budget constraints are 3. How the clinical staff operates and their workflow 4. The history and concerns of local patients.

Figure 1.3: Percent of time spent by data scientists

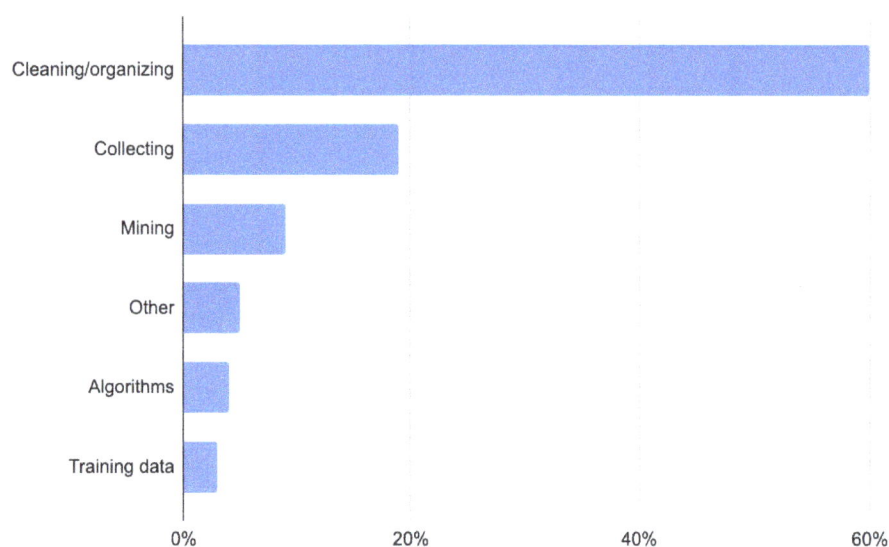

This book uses the terms data preparation and exploration, but some would simply include these processes under "exploratory data analysis" (EDA), a term proposed by John Tukey in 1977. (5) Others might use the terms "data wrangling" or "data munging" for data preparation and exploration.

It should be noted that more and more we are seeing new programs dedicated to data preparation and exploration. For example, OpenRefine is an open-source web-based program started by Google that is focused on cleaning large datasets. (6) VIDEO (7) Trifacta is a free and commercial program with the same focus. (8) VIDEO (9)

TEXTBOOK TOOLS

In this textbook, data preparation and exploration will be elucidated using real healthcare datasets and multiple tools. Spreadsheets, biostatistics, and programming languages are discussed in more detail in Chapters 2, 3, and 8 in Introduction to Biomedical Data Science. Data will be prepared, explored, and visualized with the following tools:

- Spreadsheets - Microsoft Excel (10) is the gold standard tool but Google Sheets (11) is also a consideration for basic spreadsheet functionality. The latter does include the Add-in tool *XLMiner* which is a statistical package for both types of spreadsheets and is similar to the Excel Add-in *Data Analysis.* VIDEO (12) Much of what we will be presenting in this textbook can be accomplished with spreadsheet expertise.
- Statistical packages - Two stats packages will be utilized in this chapter, jamovi (13) and BlueSky Statistics (14). Both are open-source and based on the R programming language. In other words, the computational engine is R but there is a user-friendly graphical user interface (GUI) on the front end. Jamovi includes the most common statistical functions, including descriptive statistics and visualization but does not include complex data prep, feature engineering, or machine learning. It does include linear and logistic regression that are commonly used for supervised learning. Jamovi is geared towards beginners. VIDEO (15) Another educational feature about jamovi is that it is associated with an excellent 4-hour 40-minute video that covers all possible statistical methods found in jamovi so it can serve as initial education or a fresher. VIDEO. (16) Also, a jamovi course is available that is broken into shorter videos for each topic.(17) BlueSky Statistics is far more complete as a statistical package but does have a steeper learning curve. It is available as a free open-source version and a commercial version. It is geared towards users with a statistical background. Both packages include a comprehensive free PDF user guide. VIDEO (18)
- Programming languages R and Python - Students often ask whether to learn R or Python. There is no easy answer, and some seasoned data scientists would encourage students to use both. As a generalization, R is more popular with those people with a statistics background while Python appeals to those with a computer science background. Both languages include packages for data preparation and exploration (19) (20). There are newer libraries/packages that make the process easier with less coding required. Examples of R programming libraries that facilitate this process include Caret (21) VIDEO (22), Dplyr (23) VIDEO (24), and Janitor (23,25). Examples of Python programming packages that also facilitate data processing and exploration include PyCaret (26) VIDEO (27), Pandas (28) VIDEO (29), and Pandas-profiling. (30) (31)

In this book the explanation of the programming language will occur in the body of the text or will appear one line above the code with a hashtag as below.

```
# import required libraries
import pandas as pd
```

DEFINING THE PROBLEM

The obvious starting point of a data science project is defining a problem and/or creating a hypothesis that is important to a healthcare organization. In the healthcare arena, this might arise from an individual or from a collaborative team. For example, it might result from a quality measure concern e.g., excessive readmissions for heart failure or a financial concern brought up by the C-suite (administration). Administration tends to be concerned in areas that impact the financial bottom line. This could include issues that reduce reimbursement, increase legal liability, or waste resources. It could also result from a clinical concern, e.g., the increased morbidity and mortality of patients with asthma admitted from the emergency room.

It is important to have a primary and possibly a second hypothesis as the team focuses on a new problem. Analyzing data without a working hypothesis can lead to "*data dredging*" which means you are on a "data witch hunt" where you mine data aimlessly. Remember the quote by the famous British economist Ronald Coase "*if you torture the data long enough, it will confess to anything.*" (32) That is not to say that the exploration of a large dataset might result in new or changed research directions.

LOCATING AND RETRIEVING DATA

One of the major challenges facing the data science research team is to find the right data in order to answer an important healthcare question or investigate a hypothesis. The data might not exist or it may exist in a format that is challenging. For example, does the desired data exist only in an unstructured form in clinician notes or radiology reports? More than likely the data are located in the enterprise data warehouse or data mart. Both clinical expertise to identify the data elements, and analysts equipped to employ techniques to query, extract, transform, and load (ETL) data from the data warehouse may be needed. It would not be unusual if the data must be compiled from multiple locations within the healthcare system and in multiple formats. The process of extracting data from various original sources to a location and form amenable to analysis is critical. (33) Pertinent data may be copied from the enterprise database to a dedicated data mart for analysis. Data scientists will spend considerable time writing SQL queries to tease out data the team hopes will answer the question posed by the client. The data might be moderate in size with several thousand rows, or very large requiring a "big data" approach as described in the Introduction to Biomedical Data Science chapter on big data.

DATA EXERCISES

In this chapter, we would like for you to download several packages to get comfortable with these programs. You will use these tools for exercises in the other chapters

1. Spreadsheets - an intermediate level of expertise is important
   a. Microsoft Excel - intermediate level for healthcare VIDEO (34)
   b. Google Sheets - full tutorial VIDEO (35)
2. Download jamovi https://www.jamovi.org/ (36)
   a. Begin by reading the User Guide (37)
   b. Watch the VIDEO on descriptive statistics (38)
3. Download the free open-source version of BlueSky Statistics https://www.blueskystatistics.com/ (39)
   a. Watch Part I and 2 VIDEOs (40)
4. Explore OpenRefine https://openrefine.org/ (41)
   a. View the first two videos located on the Home page
   b. We encourage readers to download and try the software
5. Explore Trifacta Wrangler https://www.trifacta.com/start-wrangling/ (42)
   a. View this introductory VIDEO (9)
   b. We encourage readers to try this software
6. Programming Languages - select one
   a. R language
      i. Download the R package. https://cran.r-project.org/mirrors.html (43) Scroll down to the USA mirrors and select one. Then choose your operating system and download
      ii. Download R Studio which is the integrated development environment (IDE) where you will do your R coding https://rstudio.com/ VIDEO (44)
   b. Python language
      i. Download Anaconda which is the popular IDE for Python https://anaconda.org/. (45) It includes the latest Python version plus almost all popular Python packages
      ii. Anaconda includes Jupyter Notebooks and JupyterLabs as the programs you will use to practice Python coding VIDEO (46)

2

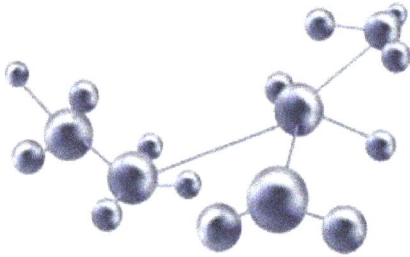

DATA PREPARATION

ROBERT HOYT   ROBERT MUENCHEN

"In God we trust, all others bring data" — W Edwards Deming

After reading the chapter the reader should be able to:

- Discuss the challenges associated with raw data
- Enumerate the most common file types encountered with data science
- Describe the important descriptive statistics used to prepare data
- Describe the data visualizations used for numeric and categorical data

DATA PREPARATION STEPS

Data preparation involves multiple early steps to clean and visualize data. It's all about "getting to know your data." As mentioned in an upcoming section, when you select a dataset you should also look for a data dictionary to provide the background, context, and specifics about the data.

In this chapter, data preparation is organized into the following sections:

1. Raw data
2. File formats
3. General inspection
4. Combining datasets
5. Reshaping datasets
6. Descriptive statistics

7. Data visualization
8. Data clean up
9. Data leakage
10. Handling missing values

Raw Data

Raw data, by definition, are messy, meaning there are errors, missing values, omissions and other inconsistencies. (21) Raw data implies that the data was extracted from a database or spreadsheet with no cleaning or error correction. This section will discuss data preparation which means the early stages of examining and cleaning the data. One of the earliest steps after retrieval is analyzing the file type and determining if the format requires conversion to a different file type for analysis. The following are the most common file types encountered in data science. Data in a spreadsheet are also referred to as columnar or tabular data.

File Formats

1. Delimited file formats:
    a. Comma separated values (.csv) - each row in a csv file represents an observation (record) and each record contains fields which are separated (delimited) by a comma. This is one of the most common file types and one that is mandated by some statistical and machine learning programs. The csv file format has several disadvantages, such as it is only capable of storing a single sheet (workbook) in a file, without any formatting and formulas. Also, if the data has strings that contain commas, you must wrap the string values in quotation marks.
    b. TAB separated data file (.tab) - are text files that contain a list of values, separated by tabs. Similar to .csv files, there is usually one record per line, with a tab between each field. TAB files can be imported into other programs such as Excel.
    c. DATA file (.data) is a data file type used by Analysis Studio that contains mined data in a plain text, tab-delimited format, including an Analysis Studio file header. Many datasets on the UCI Data Repository are in that format when downloaded. (47) The easiest remedy to convert them is to a more common format is to change the suffix to .txt, import it into Excel and export as a .csv file.
2. Microsoft Excel spreadsheet (.xls) - are older Microsoft Excel workbook files (1997-2003).
3. Microsoft Excel Open XML spreadsheet (.xlsx) - later Excel versions (2007) used the XLSX extension that contains all the information from the worksheets in a workbook, including formatting, charts, images, formulas, etc. This format is capable of handling more complex data. (10)

4. JavaScript Object Notation (.json) - is a minimal, readable format for structured data, used primarily to transmit data between a server and a web application, as an alternative to XML. (48)
5. Other - some organizations make data files available as a statistical package file, instead of a .csv or .xlsx file. For example, NHANES makes data available for export as a SAS .xpt file. (49) There is a Windows OS converter only for this file type. There is no Mac version, but jamovi accepts this file type for uploading.
6. Database files - refer to the chapter on databases in Introduction to Biomedical Data Science.
7. Web-based data - you may be able to access online data with a simple download or API, but for others you may have to "scrape" the data.
   a. There are web scrapers such as Data Miner that can pull a variety of data from web pages into a .csv or .xlsx file (50)
   b. R programming - its read.csv function can read datasets from URLs directly, and the rvest package is very popular for web page scraping.
   c. Python - you can use Pandas to read html files or use the package Beautiful Soup. (51)

In addition to the routine text format, there are occasional instances when a text file is not ASCII formatted. ASCII includes the most commonly used letters and symbols used in the US but excludes some used in Europe. (52) This is why Unicode evolved in the late 1980s and is now recognized by all computing platforms. The most common Unicodes are UTF-8 (53) and UTF-16. An online converter is available to convert ASCII text to UTF- 8. (54)

General Inspection

The next step would be a general inspection of the data. For educational purposes, we will be using the heart disease prediction dataset that can be downloaded from Data World (55) with a data dictionary or explanation of the variables in this article. (56) It is a relatively small dataset of 270 patients, with 14 columns and very few missing values, which is unrealistic. On the other hand, the dataset is relatively easy to understand, fast to analyze and it has been used for teaching machine learning for many years. Here are some early questions:

1. How many rows and columns in the dataset?
2. What are the data types - numerical, categorical, etc.?
3. Is there a header line with variable names to explain each column?
4. Is there a codebook or data dictionary?
5. What is the class (target or outcome) variable?
6. What do the descriptive statistics show?
   a. Do the minimum and maximum values make sense?
   b. What is the distribution of each numerical variable? Normal? Skewed?
   c. Are there outliers?
   d. If you have a column with the same values, can you delete it?

e. Is there a variable scale problem?
7. If you will be using machine learning to analyze, do you need to label encode categorical data? For example: heart disease = 1, no heart disease = 0. For variables with only two classes, coding them zero and one has the mathematical advantages over coding them with other values, such as 1 and 2. Traditionally, the minority class is labeled 1 and the majority class is labeled 0 in binary classification.

Combining Datasets

Data often arrives from multiple sources and must be combined before further analysis can take place. Datasets are typically combined in two ways.

1. Stacking, also known as appending or adding cases (database administrators may refer to it as a union. The datasets involved have the same variables, or nearly so. If a dataset is missing a variable, then the stacking process adds missing values for all the records from that set. Depending on the tool you use, you may be able to stack dozens of datasets at a time.
2. Joining, or merging adds additional variables to a dataset that has the same rows, or mostly the same rows. For example, a clinical trial might measure patients at three different times, so care would be taken to match the rows by patient ID.

R Code

To stack independent sets of patients:

```
library("tidyverse")
both_sexes <- bind_rows(females, males)
```

To join sets of the same patients measured before and after a treatment:

```
library("tidyverse")
both_times <- merge(before, after)
```

Reshaping Datasets

Reshaping, aka restructuring or pivoting, is often needed to convert from "wide" format to "long." Wide-format datasets have rows that contain all values per observation (e.g., patient) which often includes the same measurements repeated though time:

```
id | gender | time1 | time3 | time3

---|--------|-------|-------|------

1  |   m    |  132  |  126  | 120
```

```
2  |   f    |   127  |   123  | 118

1  |   m    |   130  |   122  | 123

2  |   f    |   131  |   124  | 116
```

Wide datasets are ideal for seeing how all the times correlate, or what their pairwise scatter plots all look like. However, this is not a good form for plotting all patient trends across time on a single plot, or for performing mixed-effects analysis of variance; the long structure is better for those tasks.

Long datasets stack all those repeated measurements into a single variable, often called "y" and puts them all along a new variable, often called time:

```
id | gender | time |  y

---|--------|------|----

1  |   m    |  1   | 132

1  |   m    |  2   | 126

1  |   m    |  3   | 118

2  |   f    |  1   | 127

2  |   f    |  2   |...
```

Since each structure has its advantages, analysts frequently find themselves switching back and forth between them, depending on the task at hand.

Spreadsheets:

Creating a pivot table in Excel (57)

Creating a pivot table in Google Sheets (58)

R Code:

From wide to long:

```
library("tidyverse")
long_dataset <- wide_dataset %>%
  pivot_longer(time1:time3,
             names_to = "time",
             values_to = "y")
```

From long to wide:

```
library("tidyverse")
wide_dataset <- long_dataset %>%
```

```
pivot_wider(names_from  = "time",
            values_from = "y")
```

Descriptive Statistics

Descriptive statistics can be easily generated by many statistical and spreadsheet programs. In jamovi (not capitalized), simply double-click or drag the variable of interest into the right upper window and it automatically generates descriptive statistics. As you scroll down to the statistics section, a user can select all of the parameters and the following figure will be generated (see figure 2.3). In addition, you can split the data and analysis by a categorical variable such as gender or the presence or absence of heart disease by dragging it to the lower window. As a result, a new table with two columns will be automatically generated for cholesterol statistics by e.g., male and female subjects. Inspection reveals valuable information such as N (number of subjects), missing data, mean, median, STD, range, min, max and quantiles. It should be apparent that the maximum is a long distance from the mean raising the issue, are there outliers? VIDEO (38)

Figure 2.3. Descriptive statistics in jamovi

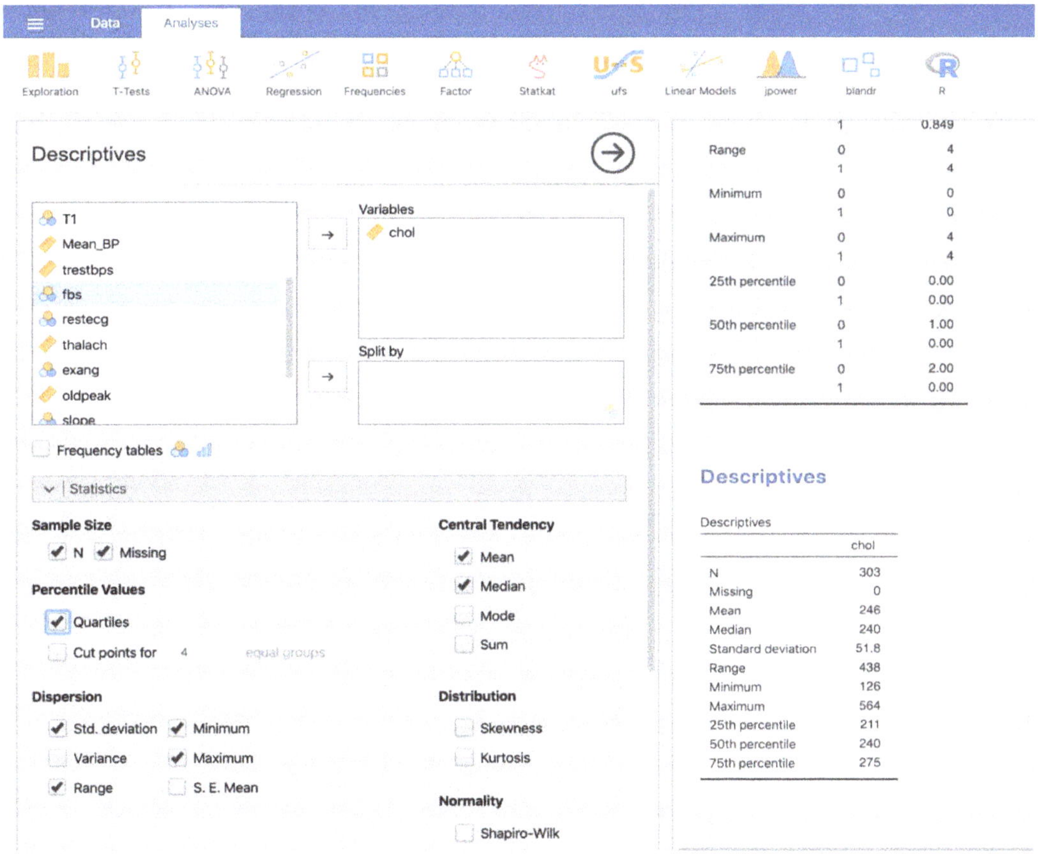

This is a reasonable starting point for most datasets, where the user examines each column to look for errors, data distribution, missing data, typos, etc. Descriptive statistics can be generated in a spreadsheet or stats package or a programming language but one could argue that a simple stats package is a very efficient approach to quickly analyze and visualize data. In addition to basic descriptive statistics, the data must pass a reality check for validity. Are the results logical? For example, are weight and height correlated in individuals? Are the numeric values within the expected range? This is where the clinicians and informaticians with healthcare domain expertise can be extremely valuable.

Spreadsheets: Excel and Google Sheets are excellent for generating descriptive statistics. Under the Data tab in Excel select the Data Analysis icon and select "descriptive statistics." If not present, the Analysis Toolpak add-in will need to be installed. VIDEO (59)The input range will need to be defined e.g., E2:E304 and an output range e.g., P2:P10 to visualize the results and it will generate the descriptive statistics there. The use of Google Sheets for descriptive statistics is very similar. VIDEO (60)

 BlueSky Statistics:
This menu item leads to a simple dialog where you select the variables to analyze:
Analysis>> Summary Analysis>> Numerical Statistical Analysis, using describe a few statistics have been cut off the right side to keep the table legible. (figure 2.4)

Figure 2.4 Numerical statistical analysis with BlueSky

	vars	n	mean	sd	median	trimmed	mad	min	max
age	1	303	54.3663	9.0821	55	54.5432	10.3782	29	77
sex	2	303	0.6832	0.466	1	0.7284	0	0	1
cp	3	303	0.967	1.0321	1	0.8642	1.4826	0	3
trestbps	4	303	131.6238	17.5381	130	130.4362	14.826	94	200
chol	5	303	246.264	51.8308	240	243.4856	47.4432	126	564
fbs	6	303	0.1485	0.3562	0	0.0617	0	0	1
restecg	7	303	0.5281	0.5259	1	0.5185	0	0	2
thalach	8	303	149.6469	22.9052	153	150.9753	22.239	71	202
exang	9	303	0.3267	0.4698	0	0.284	0	0	1
oldpeak	10	303	1.0396	1.1611	0.8	0.8556	1.1861	0	6.2
slope	11	303	1.3993	0.6162	1	1.4609	1.4826	0	2
ca	12	303	0.7294	1.0226	0	0.5391	0	0	4
thal	13	303	2.3135	0.6123	2	2.358	0	0	3
target	14	303	0.5446	0.4988	1	0.5556	0	0	1

R Language:

R offers many ways to get summary statistics. Here is the code written by BlueSky Statistics. It yields the same output, though in R, it displays using an unformatted Courier font. VIDEO (61)

```
library(psych)
describe(heart)
```

Python:

Descriptive statistics are easily performed in Python after inputting the csv file, importing the pandas package and then by the code "dataset.shape." or "df.shape" where df stands for dataframe. In this case, our data has been imported and given the label "heart" so the code is "heart.shape." Each column should be evaluated to confirm the type of variables - continuous, categorical, etc. With Python, this is accomplished by using pandas and the code "heart.dtypes" usually showing int64 (integer), float64 (decimal), and object (string). (See figure 2.5) VIDEO (62)

Figure 2.5 Python "shape" and "dtypes" methods

```
Import pandas as pd
heart = pd.read_csv('heart_disease_prediction.csv')
heart.shape
(270, 14)

  heart.dtypes

  Age                        int64
  Sex                        int64
  Chest pain type            int64
  BP                         int64
  Cholesterol                int64
  FBS over 120               int64
  EKG results                int64
  Max HR                     int64
  Exercise angina            int64
  ST depression            float64
  Slope of ST                int64
  Number of vessels fluro    int64
  Thallium                   int64
  Heart Disease             object
  dtype: object
```

The first five rows can be viewed by the code "heart.head()" as shown in figure 2.6. More rows can be visualized by inserting e.g., 10 inside the parentheses. Heart.tail() would by default display the last 5 rows.

Figure 2.6 "Head" method

```
heart.head()
```

	Age	Sex	Chest pain type	BP	Cholesterol	FBS over 120	EKG results	Max HR	Exercise angina	ST depression	Slope of ST	Number of vessels fluro	.
0	70	1	4	130	322	0	2	109	0	2.4	2	3	
1	67	0	3	115	564	0	2	160	0	1.6	2	0	
2	57	1	2	124	261	0	0	141	0	0.3	1	0	
3	64	1	4	128	263	0	0	105	1	0.2	2	1	
4	74	0	2	120	269	0	2	121	1	0.2	1	1	

Using the Python pandas function "heart.describe()" will output the count, mean, standard deviation (std), min, max of data in each column. Figure 2.7 displays the describe function.

Figure 2.7 Python "describe" method

```
heart.describe()
```

	Age	Sex	Chest pain type	BP	Cholesterol	FBS over 120	EKG results
count	270.000000	270.000000	270.000000	270.000000	270.000000	270.000000	270.000000
mean	54.433333	0.677778	3.174074	131.344444	249.659259	0.148148	1.022222
std	9.109067	0.468195	0.950090	17.861608	51.686237	0.355906	0.997891
min	29.000000	0.000000	1.000000	94.000000	126.000000	0.000000	0.000000
25%	48.000000	0.000000	3.000000	120.000000	213.000000	0.000000	0.000000
50%	55.000000	1.000000	3.000000	130.000000	245.000000	0.000000	2.000000
75%	61.000000	1.000000	4.000000	140.000000	280.000000	0.000000	2.000000
max	77.000000	1.000000	4.000000	200.000000	564.000000	1.000000	2.000000

The code "heart.info()" provides the following summary information: column data types and the number of non-null (not missing) values in each column. Figure 2.8 displays the "info" method. Note that info includes datatypes plus the number of rows per column and if there is missing data.

Figure 2.8 Python info method

```
heart.info()

<class 'pandas.core.frame.DataFrame'>
RangeIndex: 270 entries, 0 to 269
Data columns (total 14 columns):
Age                        270 non-null int64
Sex                        270 non-null int64
Chest pain type            270 non-null int64
BP                         270 non-null int64
Cholesterol                270 non-null int64
FBS over 120               270 non-null int64
EKG results                270 non-null int64
Max HR                     270 non-null int64
Exercise angina            270 non-null int64
ST depression              270 non-null float64
Slope of ST                270 non-null int64
Number of vessels fluro    270 non-null int64
Thallium                   270 non-null int64
Heart Disease              270 non-null object
dtypes: float64(1), int64(12), object(1)
memory usage: 29.7+ KB
```

Data Visualization

One of the most important steps towards understanding your dataset is visualizing it, along with descriptive statistics. Chapter 4 in the Introduction to Biomedical Data Science textbook covers data visualization but this section details the use of visualization techniques as part of data preparation and exploration. The iterative use of visualization techniques, transforming or recoding variables into new calculated or classified variables, metric development, and repeated statistical modeling can advance knowledge and create a more nuanced understanding of the dataset.

Univariate analysis (one variable): a histogram is valuable to examine numerical data, as it displays the distribution and outliers if they are present. Similarly, a density plot will also show the distribution. A box plot is also valuable to examine numerical data and plot the minimum, first quartile, second quartile (median), third quartile, and maximum. It displays outliers above or below its "whiskers." Figures 2.9, 2.10, and 2.11 demonstrate those graphs and were generated in jamovi by going to Analysis >> Exploration >> Descriptive Statistics >>Plots. All three plots show outliers. VIDEO (63)

Figure 2.9 Cholesterol histogram

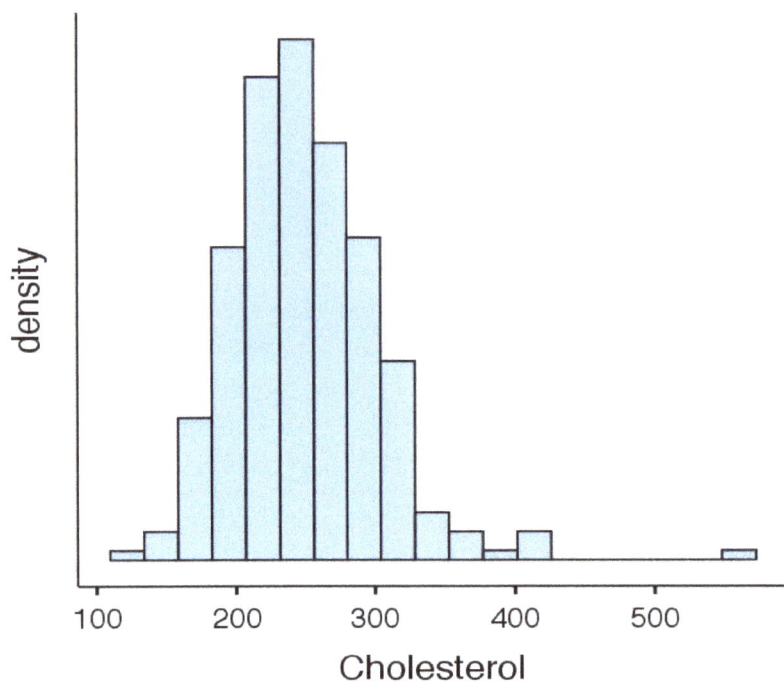

Figure 2.10 Cholesterol density distribution

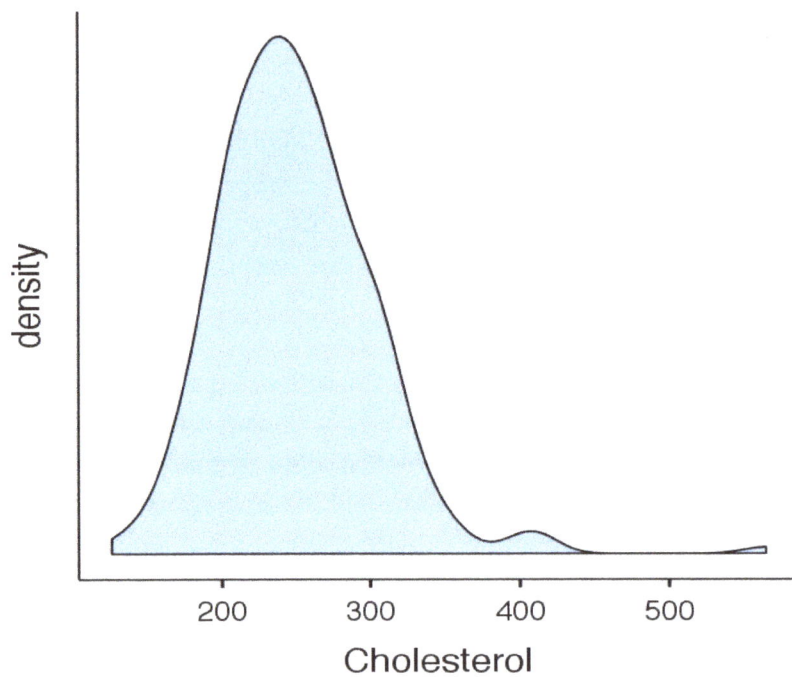

Figure 2.11 Cholesterol box plot

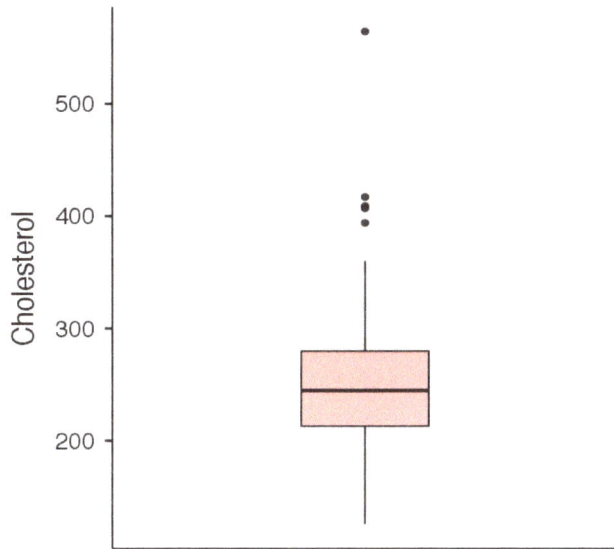

A count plot can be performed on categorical data to provide a bar graph. Note, that unlike the histogram, the columns are not touching each other. This graph clearly shows that most patients had no calcified coronary arteries on fluoroscopy (figure 2.12). Calcified coronary arteries are likely to indicate coronary disease, but the majority of patients had no calcified arteries. VIDEO (64)

Figure 2.12 Bar plot of the number of calcified blood vessels on fluoroscopy

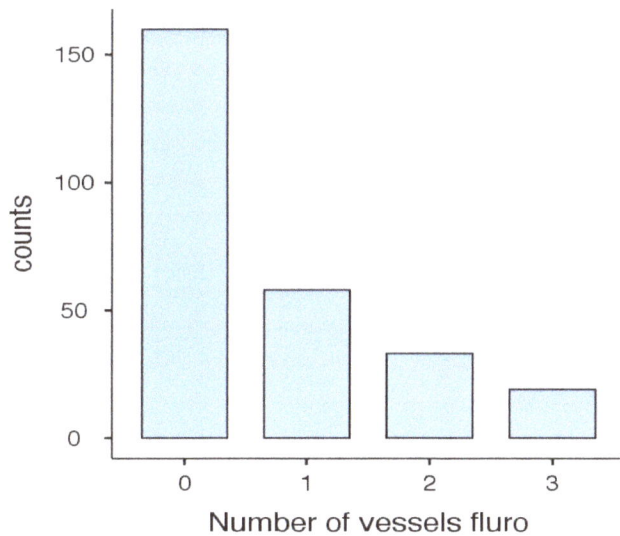

Spreadsheets: There are several ways to create a histogram and box plot in Excel but the easiest method is to highlight the data in e.g., the cholesterol column, then go to the insert menu, and select the type of chart you desire. Adding the axis labels and legend can be accomplished by selecting the Add Chart Element icon. VIDEO (65)

BlueSky Statistics:
Analysis>> Summary Analysis>> Explore Dataset (output is the same as for R below)

R Language:
```
library(summarytools);
dfSummary(heart, graph.col=TRUE) VIDEO (66)
```

Figure 2.13 Summary statistics using BlueSky

No	Variable	Stats / Values	Freqs (% of Valid)	Graph	Valid	Missing
1	age [numeric]	Mean (sd) : 54.4 (9.1) min < med < max: 29 < 55 < 77 IQR (CV) : 13 (0.2)	41 distinct values		270 (100%)	0 (0%)
2	sex [numeric]	Min : 0 Mean : 0.7 Max : 1	0: 87 (32.2%) 1: 183 (67.8%)		270 (100%)	0 (0%)
3	chest_pain_type [numeric]	Mean (sd) : 3.2 (1) min < med < max: 1 < 3 < 4 IQR (CV) : 1 (0.3)	1: 20 (7.4%) 2: 42 (15.6%) 3: 79 (29.3%) 4: 129 (47.8%)		270 (100%)	0 (0%)
4	bp [numeric]	Mean (sd) : 131.3 (17.9) min < med < max: 94 < 130 < 200 IQR (CV) : 20 (0.1)	47 distinct values		270 (100%)	0 (0%)
5	cholesterol [numeric]	Mean (sd) : 249.7 (51.7) min < med < max: 126 < 245 < 564 IQR (CV) : 67 (0.2)	144 distinct values		270 (100%)	0 (0%)
6	fbs_over_120 [numeric]	Min : 0 Mean : 0.1 Max : 1	0: 230 (85.2%) 1: 40 (14.8%)		270 (100%)	0 (0%)
7	ekg_results [numeric]	Mean (sd) : 1 (1) min < med < max: 0 < 2 < 2 IQR (CV) : 2 (1)	0: 131 (48.5%) 1: 2 (0.7%) 2: 137 (50.7%)		270 (100%)	0 (0%)
8	max_hr [numeric]	Mean (sd) : 149.7 (23.2) min < med < max: 71 < 153.5 < 202 IQR (CV) : 33 (0.2)	90 distinct values		270 (100%)	0 (0%)

Python:

Multiple histograms can be created with this simple code

```
heart.hist (figsize = (14,14)).
```

This results in the following figure 2.14 that shows several variables. VIDEO (67)

Figure 2.14. Histograms for numerical values, bar plots for categorical data

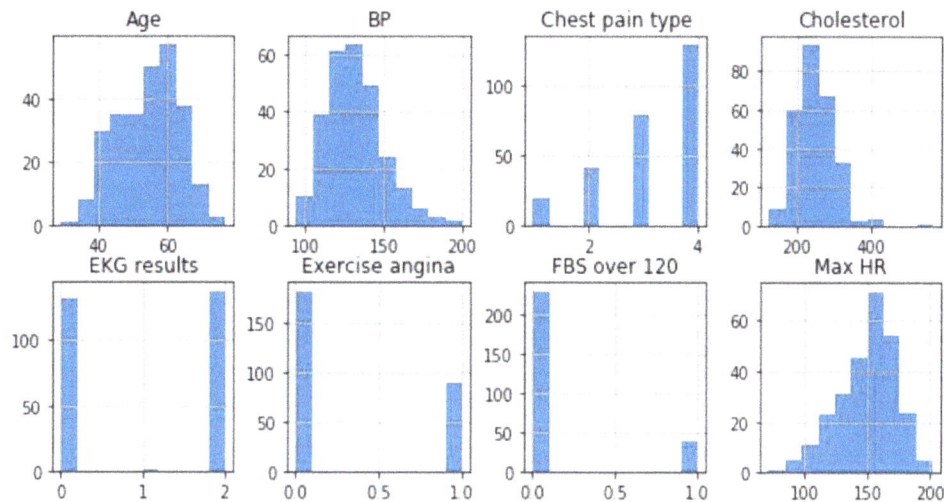

Bivariate analysis compares two variables for the strength of the association. Below is a simple 2 variable scatter plot of cholesterol and age created in jamovi (figure 2.15). This is useful as it shows increasing cholesterol levels with age.

Figure 2.15 Scatter plot of cholesterol and age

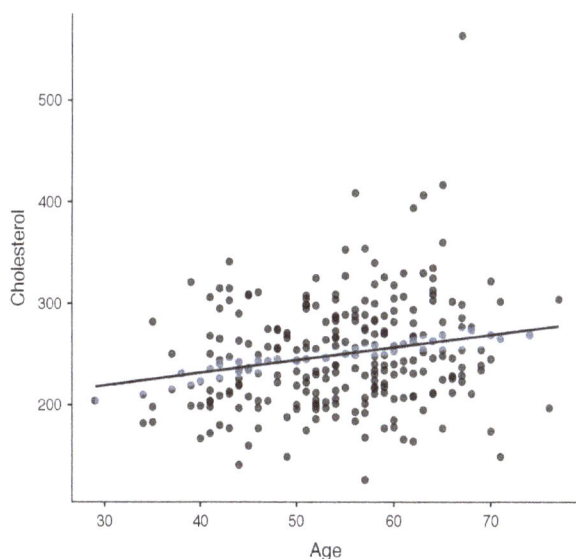

Pair plots compare multiple pairs, looking for positive or negative correlations. Below is a sample of pair plots based on the heart disease prediction data. (figure 2.16) This was created using the Python visualization library "seaborn." (68) VIDEO (69)

#import visualization package seaborn

```
Import seaborn as sns
```

#get pair plots and color based on presence or absence of heart disease

```
sns.pairplot(heart, hue = 'Heart Disease')
```

Figure 2.16 Python and Seaborn Pairwise plots

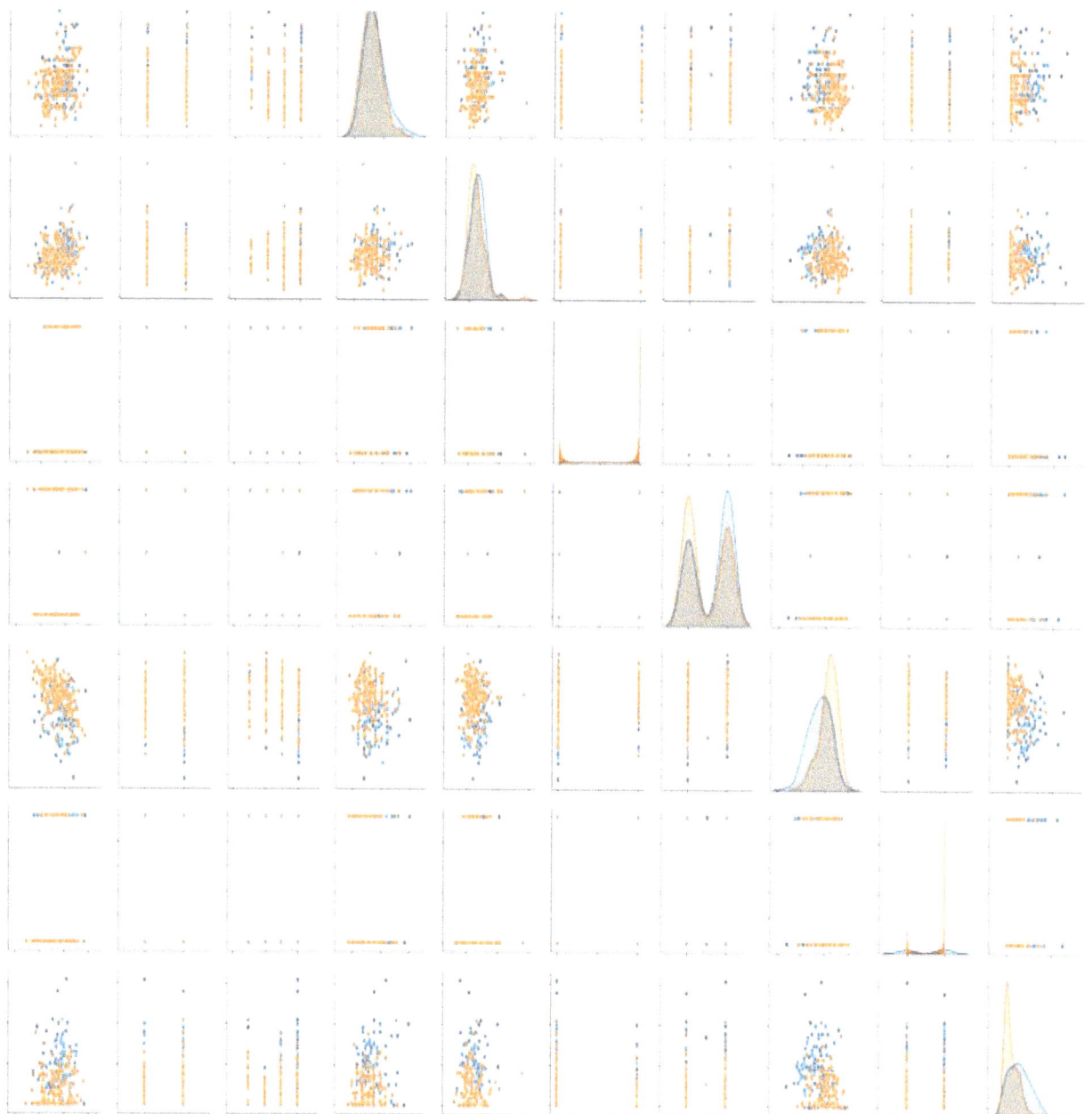

This is R's version of a similar display, done using:

```
heart %>%
  dplyr::select(age,thalach,oldpeak,slope) %>%
  ggpairs() VIDEO (70)(figure 2.17)
```

Figure 2.17 Pairwise plot using R

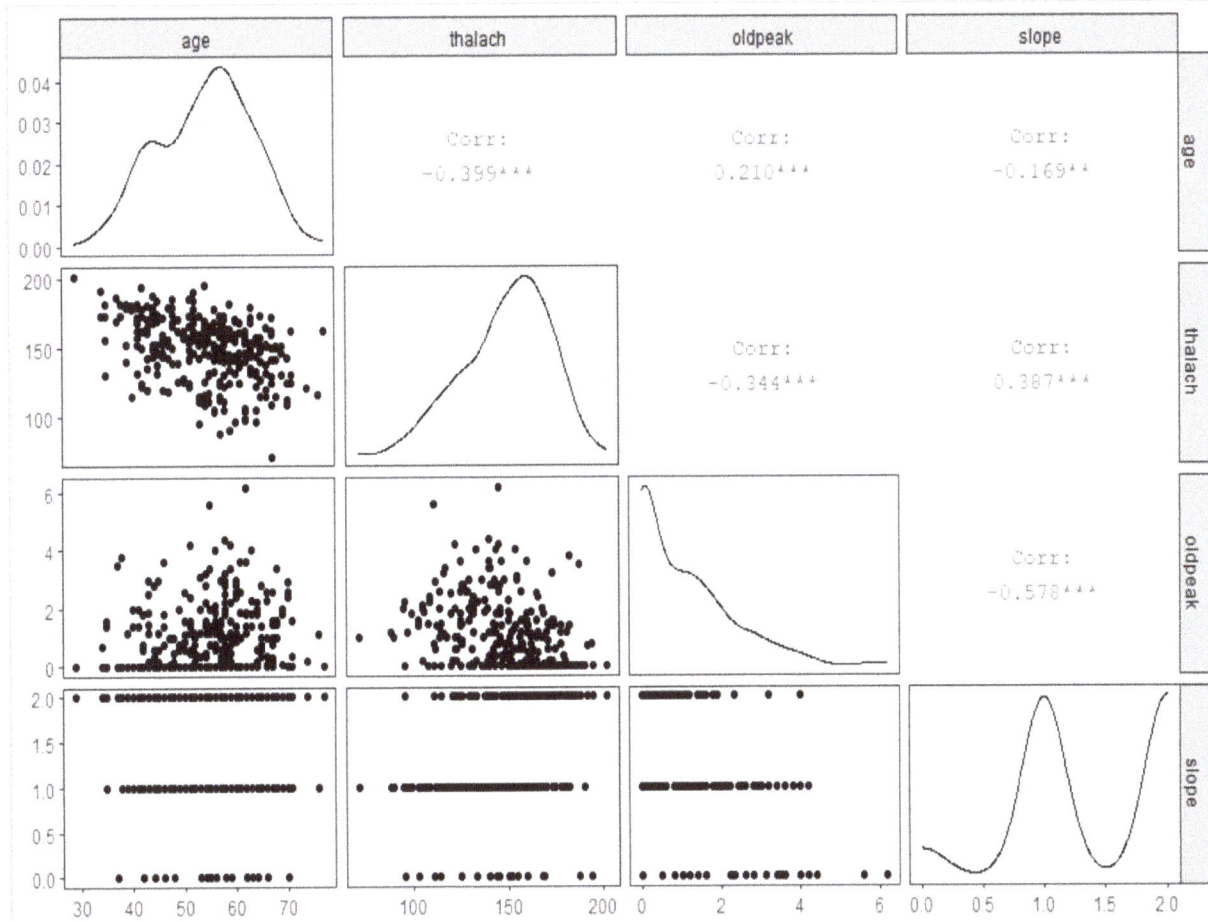

Heat Maps
Many analytical programs and programming languages will create visualizations comparing all numerical values, looking for positive or negative associations.

Spreadsheet
Select (highlight) the data and then select conditional formatting. The next step is to scroll down and select "color scales." Select the scale with green at the top and red at the bottom. Now the highlighted data will be color-coded with green for the highest values and red for the lowest. VIDEO (71) A correlation matrix is a little more complex and includes the positive and negative correlations for each relationship. VIDEO (72)

BlueSky Statistics

Analysis>> Correlation>> CorrelationTest, multi-variable>> Visualize Correlation Matrix

Figure 2.18 Color coded correlation matrix (heatmap) in BlueSky

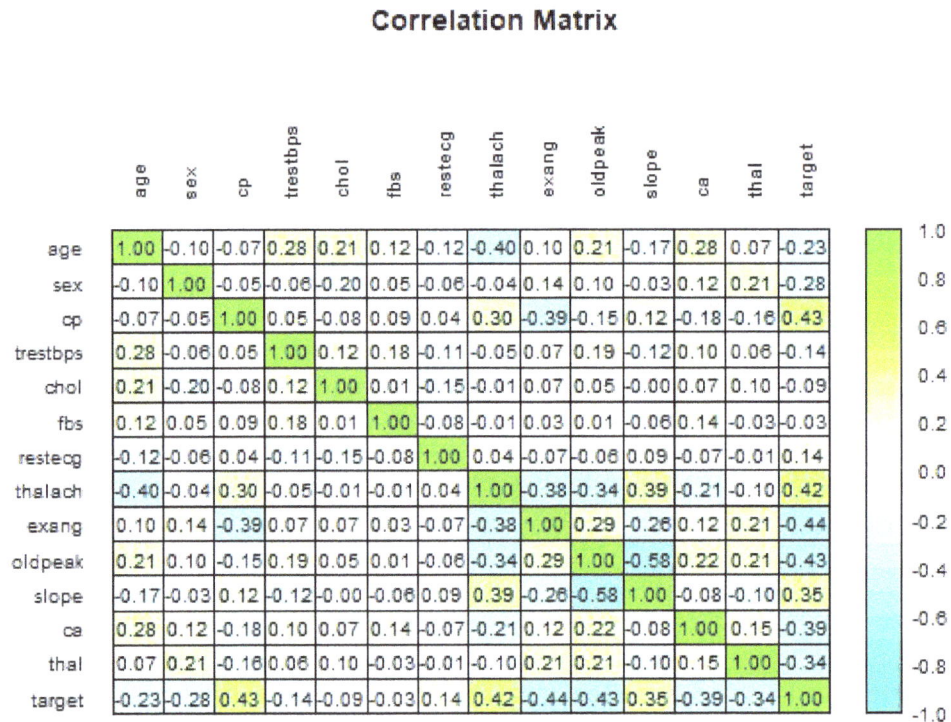

Correlation Matrix

BobMu/2020-07-22

R

This code creates the same output as BlueSky Statistics, except for the color of shading:

```
library(DescTools)
m <- heart %>% cor()
PlotCorr(m)
```

Python

Heatmap

Because there is already a heatmap based on R programming we will show the Python code but not the image. (68) VIDEO (73)

import libraries

```
import pandas as pd
```

```
import numpy as np
import seaborn as sns
import matplotlib.pyplot as plt
plt.figure(figsize=(10,5)
sns.heatmap(heart.corr(),annot=True)
```

Data Cleanup

It would be highly unusual if a large spreadsheet or dataset did not have a variety of issues that need to be addressed before analysis can occur. For example, spreadsheets might have entries labeled "NaN" which stands for "not a number."(74) The reality is that the entry was intended to be numerical but if numbers are stored as strings or if the mathematical calculation is not possible, such as dividing a number by zero, NaN can occur. One of the Excel techniques to convert strings to numbers uses the Value function. (75) Further examples of issues to consider:

- Consistent data entry: Male, M or m may be present
- If data are not stored in a consistent case, variables should all be converted to the same case after they are read in so that, e.g., "filter(sex == 'male')" does not ignore those stored as "Male" or "MALE".
- In the header, column names should not have spaces, such that systolic BP should be sysbp or sys_bp. Several software programs, e.g., WEKA will not accept spaces in the headers for csv files
- Leading or trailing blanks should be stripped out as the data are read in. This prevents logical mismatches where, for example, "filter(sex == "male") doesn't find males with even a single training blank space in its value.
- Typos - look for misspelling and other inconsistencies
- Remember that zero is not the same as a missing value. Zero is a continuous number and could affect the computation.
- Date format - convert to format used by the software or programming language. Note that many countries use (dd/mm/yyyy) whereas the US uses (mm/dd/yyyy). The most universal standard is (yyyy/mm/dd).
- Get rid of extraneous symbols: $,£, commas in numbers (1000 and not $1,000).
- Commas vs. Periods: Be aware many countries use a comma, not period as decimals.

Data Leakage

An often overlooked area of machine learning is the tendency for the training data to have inappropriate access to test data that will influence the modeling results. This is known as "data leakage." All data preparation steps such as variable selection, feature engineering imputation, and the like, should be done on the training dataset *only*. Some of these steps will result in an overly optimistic outcome on the test dataset. For example, if variables that are poor predictors are eliminated using all the data, then the model is fitted on the training data, the resulting model will do better than it ought to on the test data because the test data were involved in the variable selection process.

While it is still commonplace to see train/test splits of datasets for validation, most authorities recommend internal validation of the training dataset by a 10-fold repeated stratified cross-validation or bootstrapping. (76) Repeated means that the entire cross-validation procedure is repeated multiple times. Stratified means that each group of rows will have a similar composition as the whole dataset. This process requires that the data preparation method is prepared and fit on the training set and applied to the train and test sets within the cross-validation procedure, i.e., the folds. (31) While not part of data preparation, we should point out that current guidelines also recommend model validation using external data, which is data that is not part of the original developmental data. External data can be from a different time frame or different organization e.g., similar hospital or clinic. (77)

Missing data

One of the earliest tasks is to determine if there are missing data, and if so, how much. The presence of missing values is so common that any data set which appears to have none should be considered suspect. The missing values may have been coded with zeros or odd values, such as -999 and, if so, will have to be converted to true missing values. Missing values must be addressed as they may affect modeling. SVM and neural networks don't tolerate missing values well, whereas decision and ensemble trees do. It is common practice to first look for a pattern with missing data:

Missing Completely at Random: There is no pattern in the missing data, regardless of the variable.

Missing at Random: There is a pattern in the missing data but not related to your outcome or dependent variable.

Missing Not at Random: There is a pattern that does affect the outcome or dependent variable. Deleting the missing values could bias the outcome.

How you deal with missing data is very important as it could affect the results of your analysis and sometimes there is not a clear solution. The following are common tactics to deal with missing data. In general, it is better to not delete observations as it may adversely affect the analysis, particularly with smaller datasets.

1. **Deletion**
   a. Listwise deletion: Delete any row containing missing values within the set of variables being modeled. If your sample size is large, and the values are missing at random, you might not lose statistical power. If you are modeling, consider running the model with and without the deleted participants.
   b. Pairwise deletion: a subject with missing data is not included in certain calculations but is in others; in other words, the subject is not deleted. This offers

the benefit of maximizing the number of useful cases. However, it also means that each calculation is done on slightly different observations. That can cause mathematical problems. For example, you cannot test the difference between two models, where one is a subset of the other when using pairwise deletion.

2. **Imputation:** substituting values for missing values

   a. Heuristics - sometimes the missing value is obvious and can be manually inputted into the missing cell. Domain knowledge may be critical.

   b. Average Imputation: Input the average/mean/median for a numerical attribute into the missing cell. This method is fast and easy but does reduce the variance of the model. This approach is usually saved for when the data set is so massive that the use of more accurate methods is not feasible.

   c. Common-Point Imputation: For a rating scale (e.g., Likert), use the most commonly chosen value (i.e., the mode), or the middle point as the substituted value.

   d. Model-based Imputation: Use of predictive models, such as tree-based models, k-nearest neighbors (KNN), or multiple-regression to estimate the missing value. Tree-based models such as random forests are particularly popular for this type of imputation since they predict well without involving much effort (i.e., transforming or standardizing the data is not required). In addition, they do not have their own problems dealing with missing values.

   e. Multiple Imputation: A problem with most imputation methods is that they reduce variability across the entire set of imputed variables. This is caused by the fact that the dataset "sees" only the variability remaining within the data, not all the outside sources that may have affected all the data, had it been available. Multiple imputation addresses this problem by making multiple copies of the data set (ten is a popular number for this), imputing the missing values using one of the model-based methods, then adding some random variability to each value. An analysis is then repeated for each of the new datasets. Then the multiple models are combined. Not all modeling algorithms handle this added complexity, but for those that do, the resulting model has been shown to be more like the population that it is estimating than other approaches.

   f. Last Observation Carried Forward (LOCF) and Next Observation Carried Backward (NOCB). These techniques may be used with time-series or longitudinal data. (78)

Spreadsheets: locating missing values can be achieved in a spreadsheet by filtering each column to see how many variables exist and if there are blanks, zeros, N/As, etc.

BlueSky Statistics:
The menu item, "Data>> Missing Values>> Missing Values, model imputation" takes you to the dialog below. This example is estimating the missing waist circumference measures in the metabolic data set using a random forest model based on age, sex, and BMI. (see figure 2.19)

Figure 2.19 Imputing missing data with BlueSky

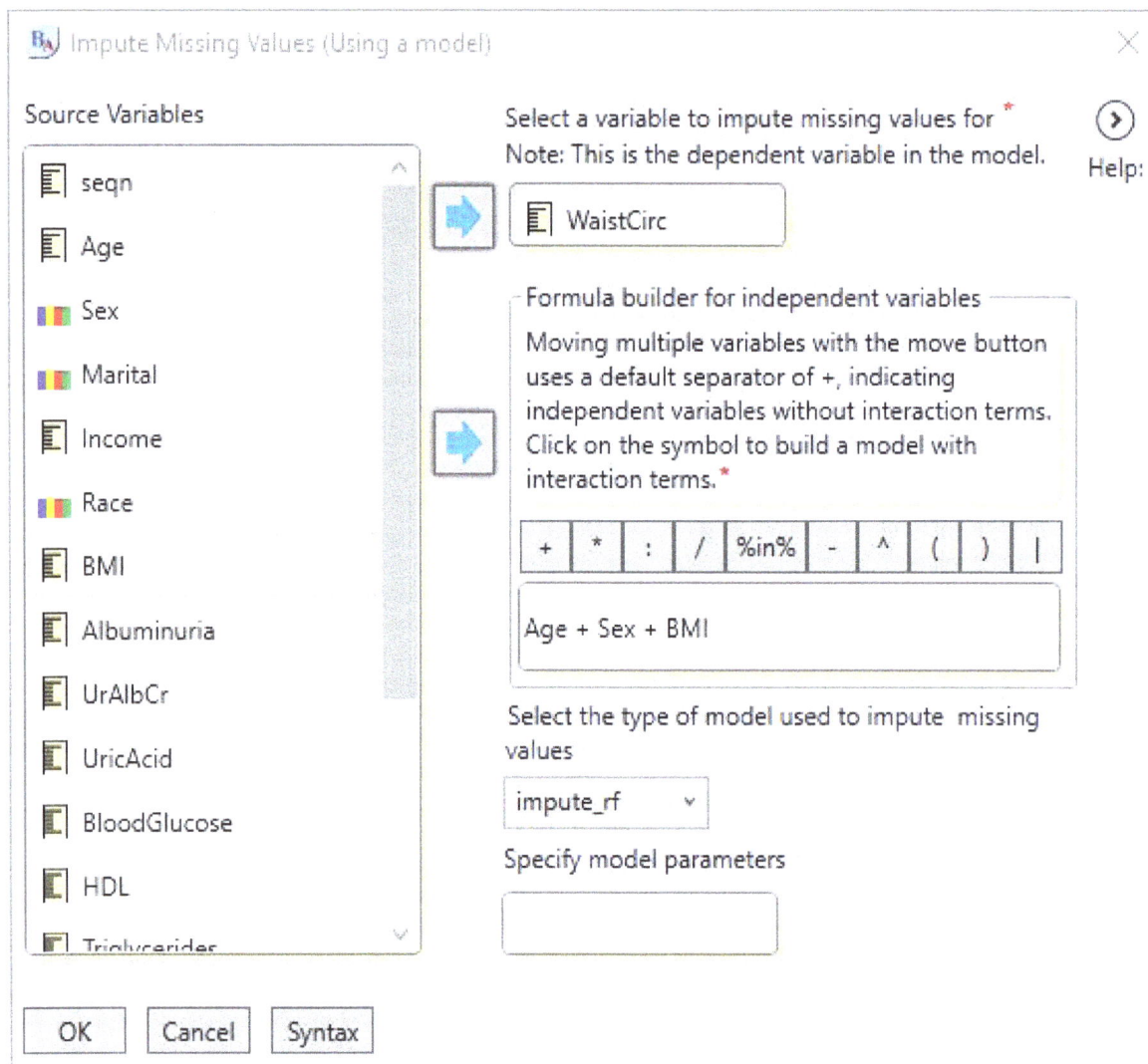

R Language: Some algorithms such as decision trees and random forest can function reasonably well with missing values. A convenient R package for missing values is "mice" which stands for multivariate imputation by chained equations. (79) The "simputation" package provides a standard way to control many other R packages, allowing it to solve most missing value imputation problems. This R code uses a Random Forest model to predict the 85 missing values for waist circumference. BlueSky Statistics wrote it based in the dialog box above. (figures 2.19, 2.20)

```
library(simputation)
metabolic$WaistCirc = impute_rf(metabolic, WaistCirc ~ Age  + Sex +
Triglycerides)
```

Figure 2.20 Imputation with R

variable	n_miss	pct_miss	n_miss_cumsum
Marital	208	8.6631	208
Income	117	4.873	325
WaistCirc	85	3.5402	410
BMI	26	1.0829	436
seqn	0	0	0
Age	0	0	0
Sex	0	0	0
Race	0	0	325
Albuminuria	0	0	436
UrAlbCr	0	0	436
UricAcid	0	0	436
BloodGlucose	0	0	436
HDL	0	0	436
Triglycerides	0	0	436
MetabolicSyndrome	0	0	436

case	n_miss	pct_miss	n_miss_cumsum
1815	3	20	174
1	2	13.3333	2
70	2	13.3333	11
131	2	13.3333	18
211	2	13.3333	22
234	2	13.3333	25
428	2	13.3333	46
510	2	13.3333	52
534	2	13.3333	55
609	2	13.3333	61

Python: It is customary to mark missing values as NaN in Python. Missing values can be labeled as NaN using the replace() function. To determine the number of missing values in each column, use pandas **info()** or **isnull()** or **notnull()** methods. The isnull() method returns a Boolean value TRUE when null value is present, whereas notnull() method returns a Boolean value TRUE, if there is no null value. Figure 2.21 shows the isnull() method applied to the Vanderbilt diabetes dataset. (80) Notice the missing values in each column. There are 13 missing glycohemoglobin levels which represent 13/403 or 3.2% missing. Depending on the goal of the project, it would not be unreasonable to delete those patients with a missing glycohemoglobin. (81) VIDEO (82)

Figure 2.21 Python isnull() method

```
diabetes.isnull().sum()

chol                     1
glucose                  0
hdl                      1
ratio                    1
glyhb                   13
age                      0
gender                   0
height                   5
weight                   1
sysbp                    5
diasbp                   5
waist                    2
hip                      2
wasit_hip_ratio          2
dtype: int64
```

If the decision is made to delete the missing values, the Python code is as follows:

modified data frame (mod_diabetes) is renamed when the missing data is deleted

```
mod_diabetes = diabetes.dropna()
```

to examine the data after the rows are deleted

```
mod_diabetes.info()
```

If the decision is to impute, use the following code:

define imputer

```
Imputer = SimpleImputer(strategy='mean')
```

fit on the dataset

```
imputer.fit(X)
```

transform the dataset

```
Xtrans = imputer.transform(X)
```

Python offers the following imputation strategies mean, median, most_frequent and constant so you can determine the best results by trying several strategies. (31)

DATA EXERCISES

1. Sign into Data World as an individual so you can access the hundreds of datasets available. https://data.world/community/open-community/ (83) You can create a new account or sign in with your Google account. At the top search window type in "*heart disease prediction*", select the blue icon which means dataset and you should be taken to the dataset. In the right upper field select "Explore this dataset." From here you can select to view the .csv file and the data dictionary. Download the data using the down arrow. Answer the following questions using a spreadsheet (Excel or Google Sheets), a stats package (jamovi or BlueSky) and a programming language (R or Python)

   a. How many rows and columns are there in the dataset?

   b. What are the data types for each variable - numerical, categorical, etc.?

   c. What is the class (target or outcome) variable? Is the outcome reasonably balanced? In other words, are there about the same number of subjects with and without heart disease?

   d. What do descriptive statistics show for each variable?

      i. Mean, median, standard deviation

      ii. Minimum, maximum, range, quartiles

      iii. Skewness, number of missing values

      iv. Split the data by Heart Disease in jamovi. Did you find differences in the predictors, when you compared those with heart disease and those without?

   e. Visualizations

      i. Look at the distribution (density plot) of each variable. Normal? Skewed?

      ii. Create a histogram and box plot for each numerical variable and a bar graph for categorical ones. Are there outliers?

   f. Create a correlation matrix using a stats package

      i. What variables had the highest positive and negative correlations with the presence or absence of heart disease? Are there predictors you should delete?

2. Try to analyze the data with as many tools as possible. Which ones were the easiest for you to learn?

3

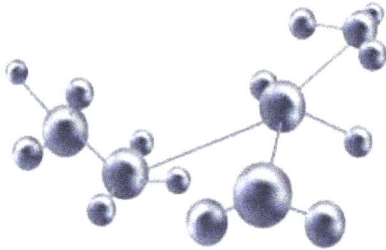

DATA EXPLORATION

ROBERT HOYT   ROBERT MUENCHEN

"Data is the new oil." — Clive Humby

After reading the chapter the reader should be able to:

- Discuss the data exploration steps needed prior to modeling
- Enumerate the differences between correlation among the predictors vs. correlation between the predictors and the outcome
- List various methods to scale data
- List different types of encoding
- Discuss the impact of imbalance datasets

DATA EXPLORATION STEPS

Data exploration is organized into the following sections. Several of the categories could be considered feature selection or feature engineering

1. Near zero variance
2. Variable correlation
3. Linear combinations
4. Duplicates
5. Outliers and influential values
6. Scaling
7. Skewness, kurtosis and normality
8. Encoding

9. Binning
10. New feature creation
11. Dimension reduction
12. Class imbalance

Near Zero Variance (NZV)

Variables that have almost no variance cannot be good predictors, so they make an easy target to remove early in the modeling process. These variables can result from filtering observations in such a way as to accidentally make a variable into a constant. For example, selecting males and keeping all variables may end up including variables like uterine cancer, yes/no. They can also result from recoding errors where, for example, two similar diagnoses were meant to be collapsed into one, but the programming logic accidentally collapsed all diagnoses into one. As you can see from these two examples, it is best to investigate variables that have no, or close to no, variance. However, among data scientists whose jobs require managing thousands of models per month, it is common to automate the elimination of such variables. Using R's tidymodels package, doing so is as simple as writing: "`step_nzv(all_numeric())`". VIDEO (84)

Variable correlation

As covered in Chapter 3 of Introduction to Biomedical Data Science, correlation measures the degree of association between two variables. The correlation squared indicates the percent of variance that it shared between the two. For example, if a pair of potential predictors correlate 0.975 or greater, then each explains 95% of the variance in the other. At some point, there is no need to have both variables in the same model since the other will add close to nothing in predictive accuracy. It should be noted that correlation does not equal causation.

Another problem caused by high correlations between predictors is that it leads to unstable predictions and inflates the standard errors of predictor equation parameters. This problem is called multicollinearity and can be reduced by eliminating one of the variables. However, correlation is not the best way to do this. A measure called Variance Inflation Factor, or VIF, can be calculated for every predictor in a linear regression equation. It measures the amount of impact each variable has on the model variance. The variable that has the highest VIF value is the one you want to remove.

Correlations can also be used to screen the data for variables to keep rather than drop. While in the previous paragraph the focus was on correlations among predictors, here the focus is on the correlation between predictors and the target (outcome) variable. Variables that do not correlate well with the target variable (e.g., below 0.01) are candidates for removal before the more detailed model training begins. However, it is critically important to do so within the training part of your training, validation, and testing steps to prevent data leakage!

This type of variable selection is called a "filter method." It is effective on very large datasets since correlations do not take much computational effort. However, screening *before* modeling is never as good as screening from within the modeling process because it only sees one variable at a time. It is possible that a variable could be eliminated that might have a significant interaction with some other predictor which would never be discovered with this approach. An alternative approach is to "wrap" variable selection into the modeling process itself. An example for linear regression is the "stepwise" process, which adds predictors one at a time to the model, then measures how well it improves the model. Measures like p-values, change in R-squared, or adjusted R-squared, tolerance, are then used to determine if the variable will be kept.

It is wise to keep in mind that any variable selection process impacts p-values for significance testing! If you generated 100 random variables and put them through any effective search process, you could expect 5 of them to appear to be "significant" predictors if you don't correct your p-values for the number of tests taken along the way. Of course, if you are holding out a test sample, those p-values will be accurate, but the holdout will have to have a big enough sample size to reach significance.

The most straightforward correlation occurs when the input and the output are numerical but there are other combinations. Here is some guidance

1. Input and output numerical - use Pearson correlation for linear relationships and Spearman for non-linear
2. Input numerical, output categorical - use an ANOVA for linear relationships and Kendall's rank coefficient for non-linear
3. Input and output are categorical - use chi-square testing which is a test for independence between categorical variables. The results of this test can be used for feature selection, where those features that are independent of the target variable can be removed.
4. Input categorical and output numerical - categorical values can be transformed to numerical so that a regression model can be used

Feature selection can be performed with programming languages but is simpler with machine learning software programs. Many of the programs generate weights for each algorithm so you can exclude those with a low correlation between the input and output and run the model again and compare performance. In addition, linear and logistic regression generate coefficients that can be analyzed. RapidMiner Go produces global correlation weights (see figure 3.1) in addition to correlation weights for each algorithm. (85) VIDEO (86)

Figure 3.1 Global weights based on correlation with target "heart disease" in RapidMiner Go

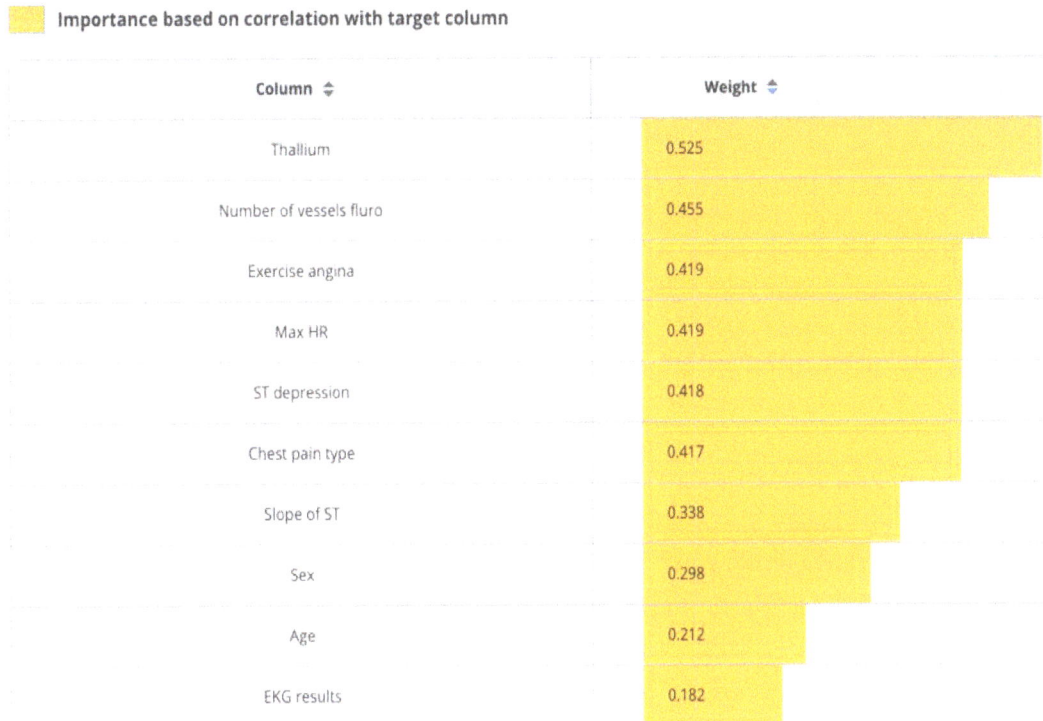

Importance based on correlation with target column

Column ⇕	Weight ⇕
Thallium	0.525
Number of vessels fluro	0.455
Exercise angina	0.419
Max HR	0.419
ST depression	0.418
Chest pain type	0.417
Slope of ST	0.338
Sex	0.298
Age	0.212
EKG results	0.182

Spreadsheets or stats packages: jamovi will generate a convenient correlation matrix as shown in table 3.1. The correlation matrix is found under "regression." This table shows several correlations between numerical variables in the heart disease prediction dataset. Note that age significantly correlates with cholesterol, maximal heart rate (max HR), and blood pressure (BP).

In Excel "correlation" in the Data Analysis program will create a correlation matrix.

Table 3.1 Correlation matrix

		Cholesterol	Max HR	Age	BP
Cholesterol	Pearson's r	—			
	p-value	—			
Max HR	Pearson's r	-0.019	—		
	p-value	0.759	—		
Age	Pearson's r	0.220	-0.402	—	
	p-value	< .001	< .001	—	
BP	Pearson's r	0.173	-0.039	0.273	—
	p-value	0.004	0.522	< .001	—

R Language:

When included in a tidymodels pipeline, this code locates correlations of 0.975 or higher and eliminates one of the pair of variables:

```
step_corr(all_predictors(), threshold = 0.975)
```

Python:

1. Python does have a SelectKBest function for feature selection that can be used. (87)
2. Recursive feature elimination (RFE) is a Python function for classification and regression that eliminates attributes that don't contribute significantly to the model. (88)
3. A correlation matrix can be created as well as a heatmap to compare numerical values. To create the correlation matrix of numerical values, the code is "heart.corr()". This results in showing the Pearson r values for each relationship, identical to those shown in table 3.2 but without p values.

Table 3.2. Python correlation matrix

```
heart.corr()
```

	Age	Sex	Chest pain type	BP	Cholesterol	FBS over 120	EKG results	Max HR	Exercise angina	ST depression	Slope of ST
Age	1.000000	-0.094401	0.096920	0.273053	0.220056	0.123458	0.128171	-0.402215	0.098297	0.194234	0.159774
Sex	-0.094401	1.000000	0.034636	-0.062693	-0.201647	0.042140	0.039253	-0.076101	0.180022	0.097412	0.050545
Chest pain type	0.096920	0.034636	1.000000	-0.043196	0.090465	-0.098537	0.074325	-0.317682	0.353160	0.167244	0.136900
BP	0.273053	-0.062693	-0.043196	1.000000	0.173019	0.155681	0.116157	-0.039136	0.082793	0.222800	0.142472
Cholesterol	0.220056	-0.201647	0.090465	0.173019	1.000000	0.025186	0.167652	-0.018739	0.078243	0.027709	-0.005755
FBS over 120	0.123458	0.042140	-0.098537	0.155681	0.025186	1.000000	0.053499	0.022494	-0.004107	-0.025538	0.044076
EKG results	0.128171	0.039253	0.074325	0.116157	0.167652	0.053499	1.000000	-0.074628	0.095098	0.120034	0.160614

Linear Combinations

A linear combination occurs when one variable is a simple combination of others. This often happens when variables and their sums are included in the same dataset. For example, numerous database columns might contain the number of patients diagnosed with each condition; then a final column might contain the total patients in the hospital. Linear combinations cause two problems. First, they simply slow down the modeling process, and for some, such as deep learning models, that can require significant additional time and money. Second, for other types of models, such as linear regression, those combination variables can make it impossible to solve. If you recall from high school algebra, it is trying to solve N equations with N-1 variables...impossible. Fortunately, the software makes it easy to discover and remove these variables. In R's tidymodels, it is done with the command "step_lincomb(all_predictors(), -all_nominal())". That searches the predictors, excluding the nominal, or categorical, ones.

Duplicates

It is quite common to encounter duplicates in large datasets which may slightly skew the results. For example, patients who spent time in the ICU may also show up as duplicates in other parts of the hospital later. Before deleting duplicates, it can be helpful to display a report of them to see where they came from. Such reports may reveal how the data collection process can be improved to prevent them in the first place. There are several methods to detect and then delete duplicates as noted in the following section.

Spreadsheets: In Excel there is a function Remove Duplicates, found under the data tab.
R Language:
These lines locate duplicate records and print a report of them:

```
library("tidyverse")
myDupRecs <- duplicated(myDuplicates)
myDupRecs
```

This line removes the duplicates:

```
heart <- heart %>% distinct()
```

Python:
calculate duplicates

```
dups = df.duplicated()
```

report if there are any duplicates

```
print(dups.any())
```

the following code removes duplicates

```
File_heart_first_record  =  file_heart.drop_duplicates  (subset  =  ["Age",
"Cholesterol", Etc], keep="first")
```

In other words, you would need to include all predictors and the "keep first" code is there so the first instance of a duplicate is not deleted.

Outliers and Influential Observations

Like duplicates, outliers need to be identified and then decisions must be made about what, if anything, to do with them. Is the outlier a mistake or extreme variance? Are there a few outliers in a lognormal distribution (see Chapter 3, Introduction to Biomedical Data Science). If so, taking the logarithm of the variable may pull them into less extreme positions. An outlier is not necessarily an influential observation. Consider a prediction of the amount of diuretic a patient was given for hypertension. You might have one patient who was extremely hypertensive, and so was given an extremely high dose, which led to an extreme decrease in systolic BP. If that person's data point falls close to the regression line of the other patients, it is an outlier, but not an influential observation. No action would need to be taken in such a case.

Outliers can be detected using a univariate or multivariate approach. As noted in the visualization section, histograms, box plots, and scatterplots can be used to visualize numerical outliers. In addition, when you transform data to z-scores (standardization) outliers will be obvious. Any value > +3 or < -3 standard deviations suggests an outlier because in a normal data distribution 99.7% of values should fall within 3 standard deviations. A distribution-free method of finding outliers is to take 1.5 times the interquartile range (IQR) or Q3-Q1, and then add and subtract it to the median. Variables outside this range are candidates for being outliers. This is done to create boxplot "whiskers" making them easy to spot.

Methods used to identify influential observations include leverage plots. Other methods based on linear regression include *dffits*, which measures how much each observation influenced the entire equation, and *dfbetas*, which show how much each case influenced each equation parameter. Most statistics packages make these easy to add to the dataset for further analysis and visualization.

If you can identify the outlier subjects then the researcher team could undertake a chart review to decide whether to delete the subject or not. For example, if the subject has always had a serum cholesterol of 500+ then this is not an error and perhaps they should remain in the study. One potential advantage of deleting an outlier would be to gain a more normal distribution which might mean you don't need to transform the variable. It is critically important that should you choose to delete any outliers in research that will be published, you must report the values you deleted and why.

Many algorithms don't function well with outliers but decision trees, random forests, gradient boosted models, and support vector machines handle outliers better than neural networks or statistical models.

Spreadsheets: Excel has a quartile function so the first step is to calculate the first quartile with a formula such as =QUARTILE(C2:C304, 1). Other steps are explained in this resource. (89)

BlueSky Statistics:
Simply choose variables in the dialog:
Graphics>> Boxplot, with MetabolicSyndrom as X, and BMI as Y, with Facets: Sex as rows (figure 3.2).

Figure 3.2 Box plot outlier detection using BlueSky

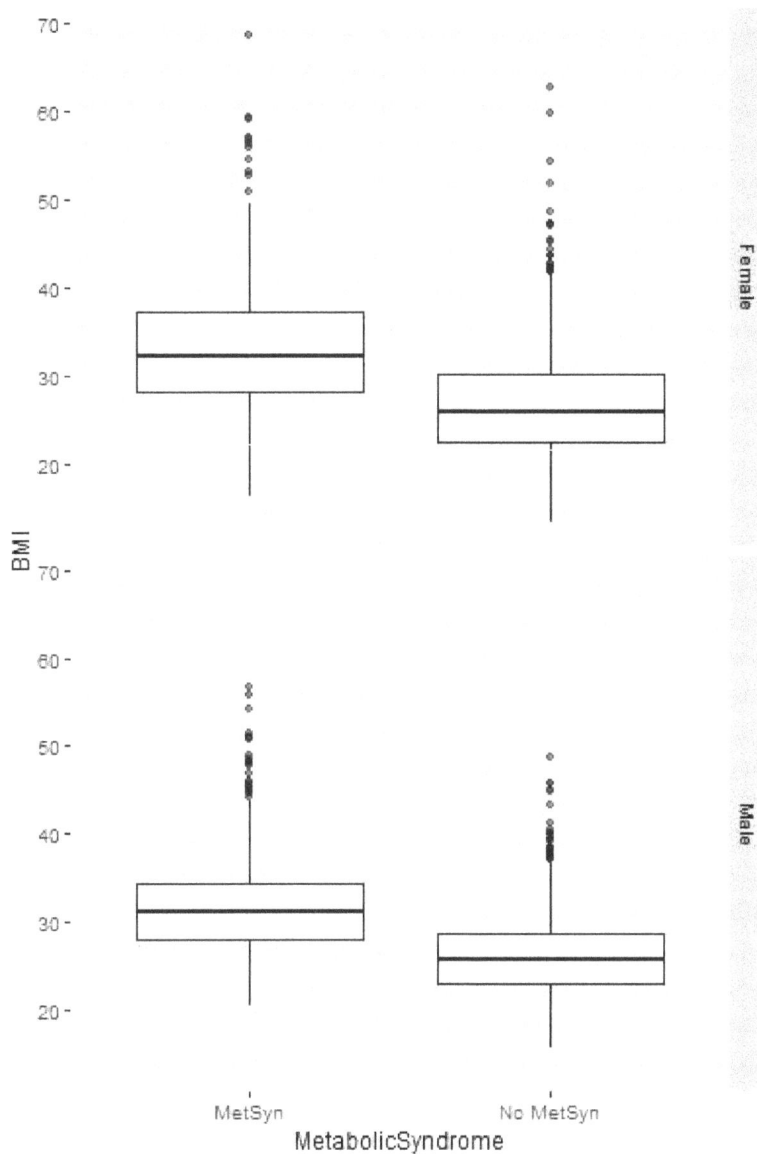

R Language:
Here is the R code to create the above boxplot. It was written by BlueSky menus, also described above.

```
ggplot(data=metabolic, aes(x = MetabolicSyndrome, y = BMI)) +
        geom_boxplot() +
        facet_grid(Sex ~ .)
```

Python: the following code will produce a box plot that shows outliers (4) above the 75th percentile (figure 3.3). A decision must be made whether these results are real and should be included or deleted. Code can be written to remove outliers based on z-score or IQR. (90)

#code a boxplot for cholesterol

```
heart.boxplot(column = ['Cholesterol'], grid = False)
```

Figure 3.3 Python Box plot

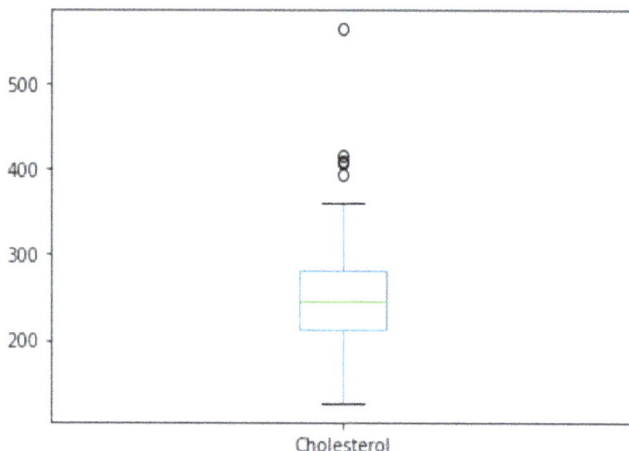

Cholesterol

Scaling

It is extremely common to have variables on different scales. For example, normal c-reactive protein (CRP) levels range between 5-10 mg/L, whereas total cholesterol (TC) is in the range of 150-300 mg/dL or about 30 times higher than CRP levels. It would be reasonable to standardize or normalize the results. Algorithms such as K-nearest neighbors, SVM, k-means clustering, and neural networks perform better with scaled data. The tree-type algorithms are less sensitive to scaling problems.

Scaling also has the benefit of shrinking the search space when tuning models, speeding the model fitting process.

The terms standardize and normalize are often used to mean the same thing. For example, WIkipedia defines them to be essentially the same. So when describing them, it's best to clarify which you mean.

1. Max-Min Normalization - to change the variable so it has a new range of 0 to 1 through the use of the formula: (x - min(x)) / (max(x) -min(x)). A slight modification to that formula limits the range from -1 to +1 for use when the original variables can take on negative values. Either approach is useful when the data cannot fall outside a given range. For example, when applying deep learning to image data, the saturation of the pixels cannot go beyond a certain range. Z-score standardization has the potential to allow values to exceed those hard limits.

2. Z-Score Standardization (aka z-score normalization) - to change the variable so it has a mean of 0 with a standard deviation of 1. This is done by subtracting the mean from each variable and then dividing by its standard deviation. While it is often assumed that transformation is applicable only to variables with normal distributions, that is not the case. However, one cannot use it to create confidence intervals unless the data are normally distributed.

Spreadsheet: standardization can be done in jamovi and Excel. In jamovi, you would compute or transform a variable with the equation *=Z (Cholesterol)*. Basically, you calculate the mean and standard deviation for a column e.g., cholesterol. If the mean is 200 with a STDEV of 10 and you have a new data point of 225, then the conversion is 225-200/10 or 2.5. The result is also known as the z-score. Standardization can be done with separate steps or Excel has a STANDARDIZE function explained in this reference. (91)

R

The tidymodels package uses this for Z-score standardization on numeric predictors:

```
step_normalize( all_numeric(), -all_outcomes() )
```

It can perform Max-Min Normalization on numeric predictors:

```
step_range(all_numeric(), -all_outcomes())
```

Python

#For standardization first import the following packages:

```
from sklearn.preprocessing import StandardScaler
import pandas
import numpy
array = heart.values
```

separate array into input and output components

```
X = array[:,0:13]
Y = array[:,13]
scaler = StandardScaler().fit(X)
rescaledX = scaler.transform(X)
```

summarize transformed data

```
numpy.set_printoptions(precision=3)
print(rescaledX[0:5,:])
```

Below is the result of rescaling multiple variables using StandardScaler (figure 3.4). This Python package StandardScaler does assume the data is normally distributed. VIDEO (92)

Figure 3.4 Python StandardScalar

```
[[ 1.712   0.689   0.871 -0.075   1.402 -0.417   0.982 -1.759 -0.701   1.181
   0.676   2.473 -0.876]
 [ 1.382 -1.45   -0.184 -0.917   6.093 -0.417   0.982   0.446 -0.701   0.481
   0.676 -0.712   1.189]
 [ 0.282   0.689 -1.238 -0.412   0.22  -0.417 -1.026 -0.375 -0.701 -0.656
  -0.954 -0.712   1.189]
 [ 1.052   0.689   0.871 -0.188   0.259 -0.417 -1.026 -1.932   1.426 -0.744
   0.676   0.35    1.189]
 [ 2.152 -1.45   -1.238 -0.636   0.375 -0.417   0.982 -1.24    1.426 -0.744
  -0.954   0.35   -0.876]]
```

Skewness, Kurtosis and Normality

Table 3.3 was created by jamovi and lists the skewness, kurtosis, and normality of serum cholesterol. Linear models benefit from data that is normally distributed, however it is quite common to have skewed medical data, particularly to the right (positive skew).

Table 3.3 Skewness, kurtosis and normality

	Cholesterol
Skewness	1.18
Std. error skewness	0.148
Kurtosis	4.90
Std. error kurtosis	0.295
Shapiro-Wilk p	< .001

A perfectly symmetrical (normal) distribution would have a skewness of zero. In that instance of zero skewness, there is no difference between the mean and median. It is recommended that you divide the skewness score by the standard skewness error. If the result is greater than 2 you should consider transformation. (13) For the example in Table 3.3 the calculation would be 1.18/0.148 = 7.9, so the data should be transformed.

One of the most common methods to transform data is log transformation. The image on the left is skewed slightly to the right largely due to outliers.(figure 3.5a) The image on the right has been log transformed. (figure 3.5b)

Figure 3.5 a Cholesterol histogram

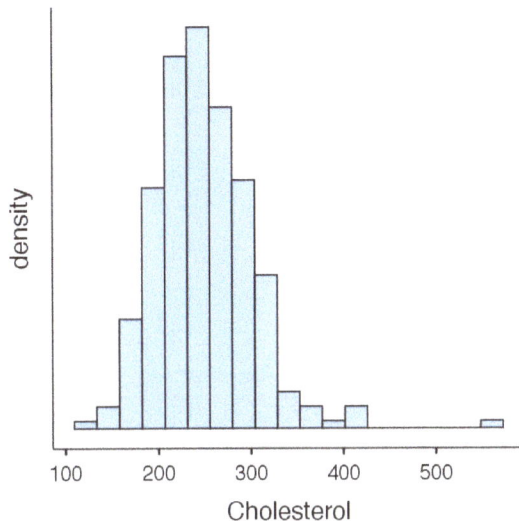

Figure 3.5 b Cholesterol after log transform

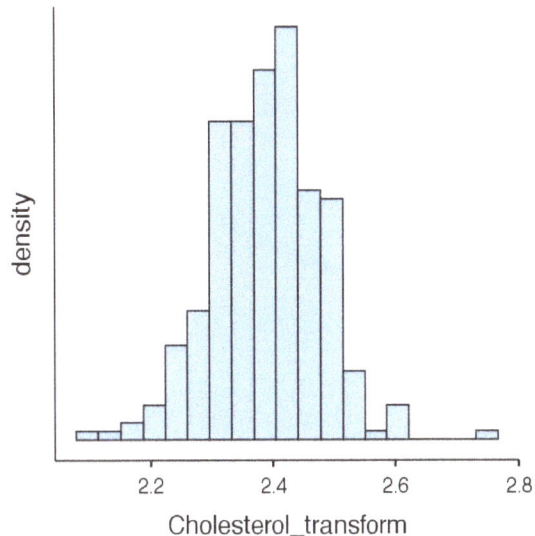

There are two methods that determine the optimum transformation to make the distribution as normal as possible. The Box-Cox transform is the oldest, but it cannot handle non-positive data. That is due to the fact that it uses transformations such as the logarithm, which is undefined for zero and negative numbers. The easiest way to use it is to call it via tidymodels' like this: `"step_BoxCox( all_numeric() )"` which applies it to all numeric variables. A more recent variation on this idea is the Yeo-Johnson algorithm. It works very similarly to Box-Cox, but can handle any numeric values. `step_YeoJohnson( all_numeric() )`

Kurtosis means the degree of "pointiness." Normal pointiness is called mesokurtic. Kurtosis is rarely used in standard data analyses.

Many statistical methods assume that the data has a normal distribution, so it is important to check. Besides visualization, there are two common ways to test for normal distribution or "normality."
1. QQ plots. The x-axis shows the theoretical quantiles, whereas the y-axis is the residuals or how far off are you from the line. With a normal distribution, it follows a straight line. Our data shows a variation in the lower and higher quantiles (figure 3.6)

Figure 3.6. QQ plot (jamovi)

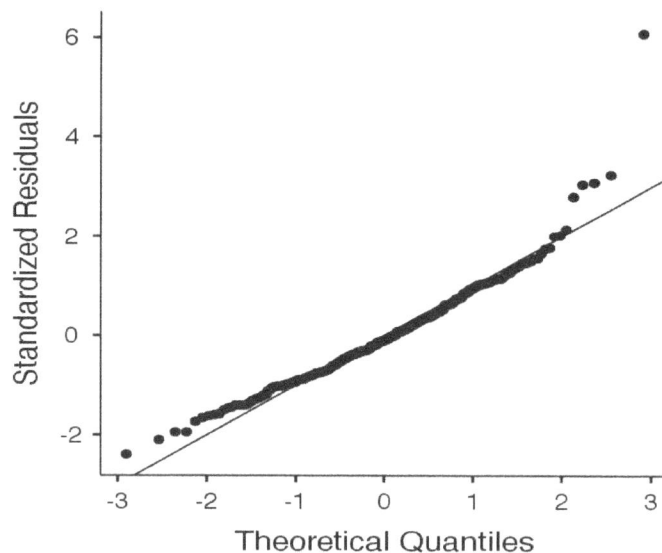

2. Shapiro-Wilk p test. We mention this test for the sake of completeness. The calculation is complicated so we will simply point out that a low p-value indicates non-normality.

Non-normal data can also affect which statistical tests you will run. For example, if the data is non-normal you should use a Wilcoxon test, instead of a routine t-test.

Statistical Packages and Excel
In jamovi go to the Data section, highlight the cholesterol column, and select transform. This will automatically create a new column that you can name. In the Fx section type = *LOG10(chol)* and the new column will display the transformed values. Using the LOG function in Excel, transformation is relatively straightforward. (93)
BlueSky Statistics
You can create histogram, density, or Q-Q plots using the following menu items:
Graphics>> Histogram
Graphics>> Density
Graphics>> Q-Q Plot

R
R's popular ggplot2 package creates histograms, density plots, and Q-Q plots using the following statements, respectively. They are also what BlueSky uses for the menu items above.

```
ggplot(data=metabolic, aes(x = HDL)) + geom_histogram()
ggplot(data=metabolic, aes(x = HDL)) + geom_density()
ggplot(data=metabolic, aes(x = HDL)) + stat_qq_point(distribution="norm")
```

Python

Log transform is one type of "power transform." Others include square root, inverse, Box-Cox, and Yeo-Johnson. All of these can be run using the Python PowerTransformer function. (94) The following demonstrates log transformation without PowerTransformer.
#First import Numpy

```
Import numpy as np
chol_log = np.log(df ['chol'])
chol_log.skew() (95)
```

Encoding

Some machine learning algorithms require numerical variables. In order to change a categorical variable to numerical, one of the most common methods is label (also called ordinal) encoding. As you can see in figure 3.7 a. multiple countries are listed. With label encoding Japan is now 0, US is 1, etc. in figure 3.7 b. One problem with this method is that it now gives order or hierarchy to the column. China has a higher number than other countries. If this was simply changing a Likert scale for disapprove to 0 and highly approve to 4 there would be no issue. Label encoding is never appropriate for analysis unless it is followed by an additional step, which tells your software that the variable is categorical.

Figures 3.7 a. Country column as categorical data

Figure 3.7 b. Country column after Label encoding

ID	Country	Population
1	Japan	127185332
2	U.S	326766748
3	India	1354051854
4	China	1415045928
5	U.S	326766748
6	India	1354051854

ID	Country	Population
1	0	127185332
2	1	326766748
3	2	1354051854
4	3	1415045928
5	1	326766748
6	2	1354051854

In order to address the issue of false hierarchy, "dummy" variable (aka indicator variable) encoding is used. This uses a series of binary variables to indicate category membership. A common example is gender. You can create a variable called "female", which has a value of 1 for females and zero for males. Note that only one variable is needed to encode two categories. This is called "leave-one-out" (LOO) encoding. You could also create a variable called "male" that has a 1 for the males and zero for females. However, that is redundant, and you could not use both of them as predictors in a linear regression equation. It would be asking it to calculate two parameters when you have given it only one variable. A key question in LOO encoding is which category to leave out. That is often the largest category. For example, a hospital in the U.S. could leave out the U.S. when encoding country of origin, since most of the patients will be from the U.S. Keep in mind we are talking about encoding for modeling, not for database design. The people who enter data on arriving patients will certainly want to see the U.S. on their data entry screen!

Some statistics software, such as R, BlueSky, jamovi, and SAS, will automatically generate LOO dummy variables whenever you identify a variable as a factor (or class) variable, and then use it in a statistical model.

The alternative to LOO encoding is "one-hot encoding" that is employed to assign every categorical value to a new column and code it as 1 if applicable and 0 if not. That is, it's the same idea, but none of the categories are left out. Figures 3.8 a. and b. should make that clear. The downside would be the creation of many more columns if, for example, you were analyzing 100 countries.

As we discussed, LOO encoding is required for the predictors in many statistical models, such as linear regression. Other model types, such as the tree-based ones, work fine with one-hot encoding. In fact, it is often easier to interpret those models with one-hot encoding because you do not have to consider the "none of the others" category yourself. Some models, such as some neural networks, require a classification target to be one-hot encoded.

Figure 3.8 a. Country column as categorical data

Figure 3.8 b. Country column data after one-hot encoding

ID	Country	Population
1	Japan	127185332
2	U.S	326766748
3	India	1354051854
4	China	1415045928
5	U.S	326766748
6	India	1354051854

ID	Country_Japan	Country_U.S	Country_India	Country_China	Population
1	1	0	0	0	127185332
2	0	1	0	0	326766748
3	0	0	1	0	1354051854
4	0	0	0	1	1415045928
5	0	1	0	0	326766748
6	0	0	1	0	1354051854

Spreadsheet
There is no option to do one-hot encoding in jamovi and there is no easy way in Excel. We recommend using BlueSky Statistics or a programming language.

BlueSky Statistics
Since BlueSky does its calculations in R, factor (categorical) variables used in statistical models will automatically create leave-one-out encoded dummy variables. However, it offers far more control about how dummies are created by choosing, "Data>> Compute Dummy Variables" to

bring up the dialog below. It asks what level to treat as "reference", which is asking which one is left out and will be indicated by all zeros on the others. Note that if you choose "keep all levels" (i.e., one-hot) it warns you that it is not recommended for statistical models. (figure 3.9)

Figure 3.9 Dumming coding in BlueSky

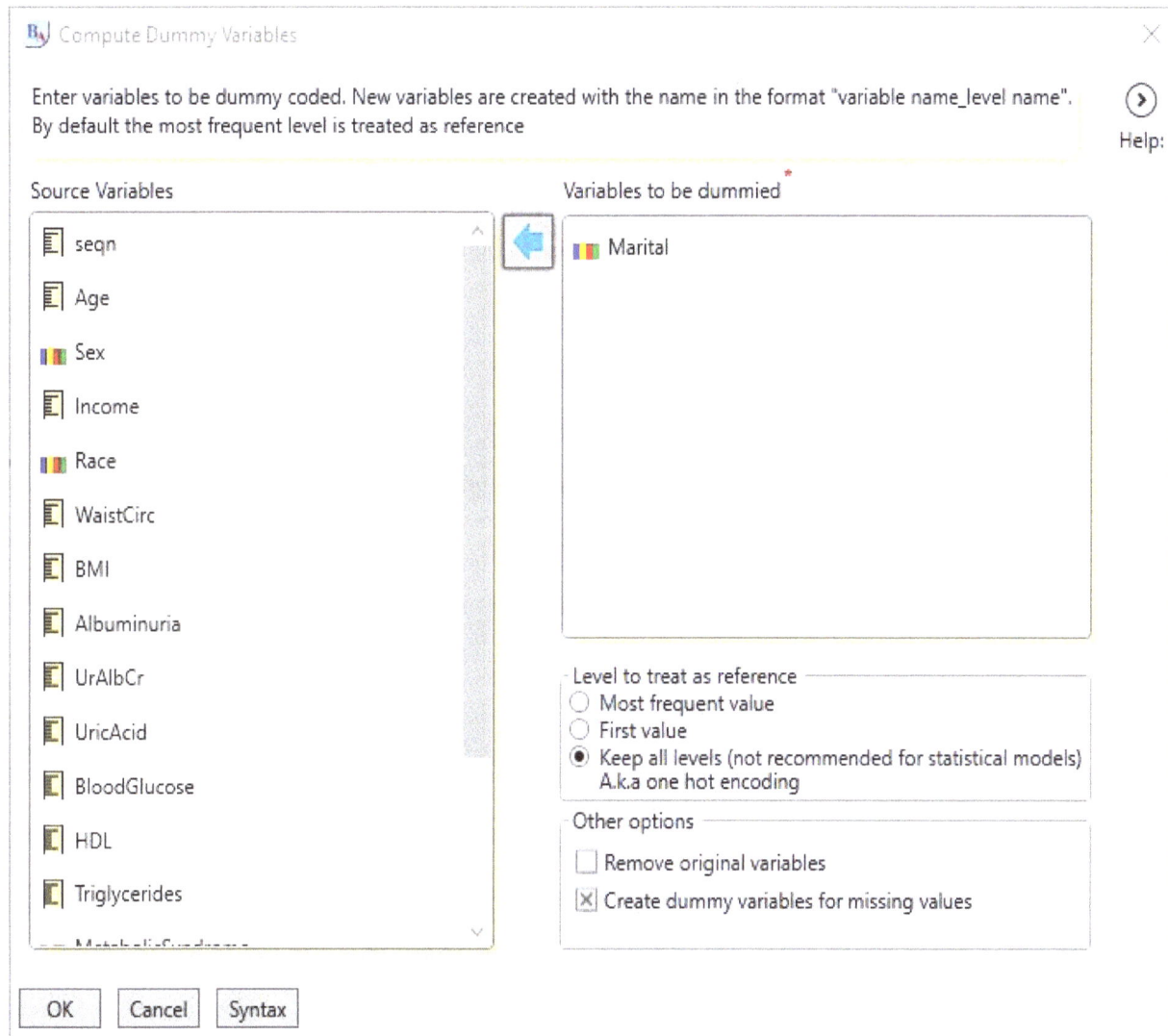

R

R's fastDummies package is a good way to create dummy variables (the BlueSky example above uses it):

```
library(fastDummies)
metabolic_with_dummies <- metabolic %>% dummy_cols()
```

When using tidymodels, this line does it. You can change one_hot to TRUE to use that type of encoding:

```
step_dummy(all_nominal(), one_hot = FALSE)
```

Python
Label encoding:
import required libraries

```python
import pandas as pd
import numpy as np
```

creating initial dataframe

```python
country = ('Japan','U.S','India','China')
country_df = pd.DataFrame(country_types, columns=['Country'])
```

converting type of columns to 'category'

```python
country_df['Country'] = country_df['Country'].astype('category')
```

Assigning numerical values and storing in another column

```python
country_df['Country_Cat'] = country_df['Country'].cat.codes
Country_df
```

One-hot encoding: Uses the pandas get_dummies function.(96)
#import required libraries

```python
import pandas as pd
import numpy as np
```

creating initial dataframe

```python
country = ('Japan','U.S','India','China')
country_df = pd.DataFrame(country_types, columns=['Country'])
```

generate binary values using get_dummies

```python
dum_df      =      pd.get_dummies(country_df,      columns=["Country"],
prefix=["Country_is"] )
```

merge with main df country_df on key values

```python
country_df = country_df.join(dum_df)
country_df
```

Binning

There are times when converting continuous data into categories or bins makes sense. For example, if you need to develop a cutoff point for diagnosis. Also, association rules are run on categorical data only. Sometimes age is converted to decade bins, e.g., 20-30, 31-39, 40-49, and so forth. This process is also called discretization. As a general rule, however, binning should be avoided for several reasons: (97)
   1. When performing hypothesis testing, binning may result in a loss of statistical power

2. The loss of information as a result of binning could simplify a histogram such that you could no longer see data trends
3. Bins could be misleading. For example, how different is the 20-30 age bin from the 31-39 bin?
4. Bins may prevent you from finding a simple linear model, such as, "for each year of age, systolic BP increases x%"

New Feature Creation

It is possible that a new column may need to be created that will include a calculated variable. For example, you have data on total cholesterol and HDL cholesterol and now want to have an HDL cholesterol/total cholesterol/ ratio. All statistics and ML/AI software makes this easy by entering formulas like HDL_ratio = HDL cholesterol/total_cholesterol.

Dimension Reduction

The "curse of dimensionality" means that as the number of predictors increases, the requirements for training data and the risk of overfitting also increases. (98) There are multiple ways to reduce the number of attributes, such as eliminating those with near-zero variance or those that are highly correlated with other attributes, as covered in a previous section. There are many formal ways to reduce the number of predictors or attributes but the most commonly used one is principal component analysis (PCA). PCA is actually an unsupervised machine learning technique that analyzes the predictors and re-groups them to simplify the model. This would be an example of "dimension reduction or data reduction." PCA can be performed by most statistical packages and ML/AI software. (99)

Class Imbalance

It is common with biomedical datasets to have a class imbalance, that is, the minority (positive) class of interest e.g., cancer has far fewer subjects than the majority (negative) class benign. In other words, in this scenario most biopsies are benign, not malignant. By convention, the minority class is labeled =1, and the majority class is labeled = 0. This imbalance causes multiple problems for machine learning binary classification. The learning process for most classification algorithms favor the majority class as there are more data samples, but ironically we tend to be more interested in the minority class. Accuracy is no longer a good performance measurement, as it is overly optimistic, a phenomenon known as the "accuracy paradox." If 5% of subjects have cancer then classifying all patients as benign would have a 95% chance of being correct. The odds of overfitting is also greater with class imbalance. The AUC can still be used but many authorities would instead recommend a precision-recall curve (PRC) instead of the AUC. The AUC curve helps to measure the performance of both classes, whereas the PRC measures the minority class. Figure 3.10 below displays a PRC on the heart dataset.

Figure 3.10 Precision recall curve on the logistic regression model (Pycaret)

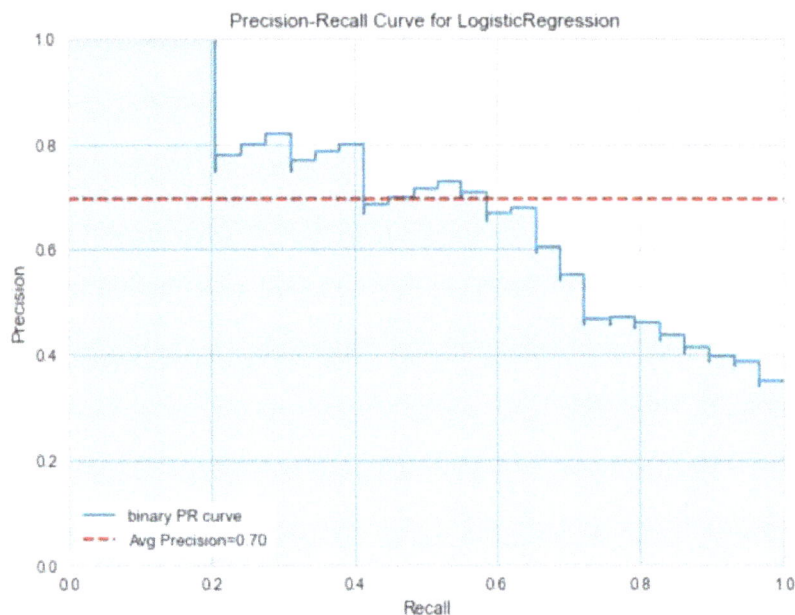

Because there are more negative than positive values, you are likely to have more false positives which, in turn, lowers precision, because precision = TP/(TP + FP). Remember that recall is important when the focus is on keeping false negatives low, whereas precision is important when the focus is keeping false positives low. As mentioned in the machine learning chapter, the F-score or F-measure is the harmonic mean between recall and precision. Scores can be from 0-1 and are calculated as 2 x Precision x Recall / Precision + Recall. Two other scores used with class imbalance are LogLoss and Brier Score. (100)

A variety of techniques are available to improve class imbalance but there is no guarantee or silver bullet. Here are the major categories of dealing with class imbalance:

1. Find more data - the most helpful, but least likely would be to locate more data so that the minority class is larger
2. Resampling - only performed on the training dataset!
   a. Undersampling - if the majority class is very large, an option would be to sample and reduce that class so the majority and minority classes are about equal. There are multiple techniques to undersample, but the simplest Python method is the *RandomUnderSampler* function. R's tidymodels package uses the function call, `step_downsample(under_ratio = 1)`. Other techniques include Tomek Links and Edited Nearest Neighbors Rule.
   b. Oversampling - this is the reverse of undersampling. The minority class is sampled, with replacement, until it is roughly the same size as the majority class. R's tidymodels package does this using: `step_upsample(over_ratio = 1)`

c. Synthetic Oversampling of Minority Technique (SMOTE) is one of the most popular approaches to balance datasets. (101) It selects synthetic examples that are close to the feature space by using the k-nearest neighbor algorithm. There are multiple modifications of SMOTE with none felt to be unequivocally superior. VIDEO (102)

d. Under and oversampling techniques - some recommend using both under and oversampling for imbalanced datasets. Examples of this combination approach include SMOTE and Random Undersampling, SMOTE and Tomek Links, and SMOTE and Edited Nearest Neighbors Rule. There is a Python imbalanced-learn library that can create a sequence of techniques in a pipeline as well. (103)

3. Over-sampling applies bootstrapping to generate new random data based on a distribution function and cross-validation should always be done before over-sampling, in order to avoid overfitting. Several authorities recommend a special type of k-fold cross validation known as "stratified cross-validation" which maintains the same class distribution for each fold as in the original dataset. Cross-validation can be run multiple times and the mean of the folds recorded. VIDEO (104)

4. Hyperparameter optimization - tweaking algorithms
   a. There are a variety of adjustments to algorithms to make them perform better with imbalanced data
      i. Weighted neural networks
      ii. Class weighted XGBoost

NOTE: There is a data checklist in the Appendix and on informaticseducation.org that will serve to remind readers about the normal steps taken in data preparation and exploration.

DATA EXERCISES

1. Sign into Data World and search for the dataset "Hepatitis and Mortality." Download
2. Open the file in Excel or Google Sheets as this dataset has several issues that need to be corrected:
   a. Create a new column A and add "ID" as most research datasets have some means of identifying patients, as they are otherwise anonymous. In the new column, first row, type =ROW (A2) then hit enter and it should insert the number 1. Drag the mark (handle) in the lower right cell corner downward to add numbers for all 155 subjects
   b. Note that there are a lot of values of (?) inserted throughout the dataset. They should be converted to blanks for the time being
      i. Highlight the columns with ?'s. Go to Edit >> Find and replace. In the find search box type in ~?. Leave the replace box blank. Note: you must have a tilde ~ before the ? in order for it to work
   c. Using Find and Replace
      i. Change to LIVE =1, DIE =0
      ii. Change to Male =0, Female =1. Always change female first because male is part of the word female.

   iii. In columns C-M Find and Replace Yes =1, No =0
3. Create a correlation matrix using a stats package or programming language
  a. What predictors had the most positive and negative correlations with the outcome "class"?
4. Using a stats package or programming language, determine how many missing values you have in each column and row.
  a. Perform descriptive statistics on the numerical value columns (4). Which one had the most missing values? Was it strongly correlated with the outcome? If not it might be reasonable to create a model with and without this variable
5. Include skewness in your descriptive statistics. Divide it by the skewness standard error. How many were over 2 which means skewed data?
6. Visualize the 4 numerical liver biomarkers with box plots, density plots, and histograms. Which one was not skewed to the right?
  a. In jamovi highlight the Alk_Phoshatase column, go to Data, select transform
  b. The formula is =LOG10(ALK_PHOPHATE), hit enter. Look at the new values for the column
  c. Go back to Exploration >> Descriptives >> Plot and select histogram and density. What do you now notice about the distribution?
7. Notice that of the four liver biomarkers ALK_PHOSPHATE is on a higher scale. Again using jamovi
  a. Go to Data >> highlight the ALK_PHOSPHATE column. Go to Transform and write the formula =Z(ALK_PHOSPHATE), hit enter. This will standardize the data in that column and create Z scores and a new column with these new values. Remember if any are values <-3 or >+3 they are outliers.
8. Impute missing numerical values for one of the numerical liver biomarkers with the median value, using BlueSky, R, or Python, as described in the chapter.

4

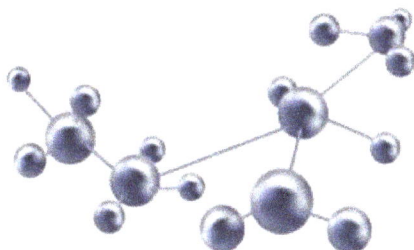

AUTOMATED DATA PREPARATION AND EXPLORATION

ROBERT HOYT   ROBERT MUENCHEN

"Without a systematic way to start and keep data clean, bad data will happen." — Donato Diorio

LEARNING OBJECTIVES

After reading the chapter the reader should be able to:

- Discuss the reasons why automated machine learning (AutoML) has become popular
- Enumerate several AutoML programming packages
- List several commercial AutoML platforms
- Understand the potential limitations of AutoML

BACKGROUND

It is not surprising that one of the most recent trends in data science is automation. This is because many of the steps in the data science process are time-consuming, there is a shortage of data scientists and there is a steep learning curve associated with learning R or Python programming languages. In addition, many consider data preparation and exploration to be mundane, so any new methods to save time are welcomed. There is also the belief that simpler systems may be particularly helpful for non-data scientists and "citizen scientists." A 2019 Survey by Gartner asked business leaders about the potential impact of augmented data science and ML and their opinion of the impact was as follows: low/no impact 7%; medium impact 26%; high impact 40% and transformational 27%. (105)

The most commonly used term for this automation is automated machine learning (AutoM), but the reality is that it probably should be called AutoDS or automated data science because we are moving towards automating the majority of the data science processes. There is no universal definition of AutoML but it is clear that the goal is to automate the entire machine learning pipeline.

Early AutoML efforts evolved from academics, early ML super-users, and later startups. One of the first was Auto-Weka (2013), followed by Auto-sklearn (2014) and then TPOT (2015) that was developed by the University of Pennsylvania. (106) One of the most successful and earliest examples of AutoML was Google Cloud AutoML. (107) Their Cloud Dataprep tool for data preparation is actually the same as the Trifacta commercial tool. (6) They use reinforcement learning to select the optimal deep learning architecture. This process is known as a neural architecture search (NAS). (108)

Neural architecture search is highly complex so newer strategies are being considered. This is a rapidly changing field with new technologies appearing and improving all the time. It is conceivable that there will be platforms that can design and optimize deep learning models with minimal human input. Is it possible new technologies such as GPT-3 can analyze the dataset or image, select and run the model and explain it? (109)

For the foreseeable future, it is clear that human intervention to some degree will be necessary for many of the data science processes. Most of the steps outlined in Figure 1 in Chapter 1 can be at least partially automated. Here are the data science steps that might be automated:

1. Automated potential
    a. Clean and prepare the data
    b. Explore and visualize the data
    c. Model generation
    d. Tune and explain the model
    e. Deploy and save the model
2. Limited automation potential
    a. Define the problem
    b. Locate the data
    c. Communicate the results

Define the problem

The first step (talking to the client) and the last step (communicating the findings) cannot be replaced by technology for obvious reasons. The initial step of meeting with the client (usually a hospital or healthcare system) is critical so there can be a bilateral understanding of what the needs really are, the capabilities of the data science team and associated technologies, and the realistic financial constraints. It is also important to discuss if there are patient safety issues, whether there is a reasonable business case, and whether there is buy-in by all relevant partners. More meetings are also likely to report progress, possibly adjust the model, locate more data, etc.

Locate the Data

Locating data cannot be automated at this time as the data is likely to be found in different formats, and in different locations. Nevertheless, as we continue to make large data repositories openly available for research, it is possible that a comprehensive AutoML platform will know where to look for data for e.g., external validation. Alternately, an intelligent platform may generate new data or images by using methods such as SMOTE or a generative adversarial network (GAN). (110)

Clean and Prepare the Data

Duplicate data can be identified and removed, incorrect formats can be corrected, missing values can be imputed, skewed data can be transformed, scalar issues can be standardized and data can be encoded as needed. Those steps have already been automated today.

Explore and Visualize the Data

Automated feature engineering involves three processes: 1. Feature selection - using algorithms to select the features that are not irrelevant or redundant, thus simplifying the model 2. Feature construction - using algorithms to create new features from existing ones. This would include transformation and standardization and 3. Feature extraction - using techniques like principal component analysis (PCA) an entirely new set of predictors is created. (59)

Because variables can be identified as categorical or numerical there is no reason appropriate visualizations can't be generated. Similarly, correlations with the outcome and correlations between predictors can be analyzed and excessively correlated predictors (multicollinearity) can be deleted. AutoML should also be able to determine if principal component analysis (PCA) is appropriate to reduce predictors and in so doing decrease the tendency towards overfitting.

Model Generation

For non-neural network machine learning programs, it is more common for a platform or programming language package to offer multiple e.g., classification algorithms and let the user select the best performing one. The difficulty is that performance should be evaluated by looking at multiple measures of model effectiveness and not just e.g., accuracy that has several limitations.

Tune and Explain the Model

Data scientists will tune the model for maximal performance by tweaking or tuning the algorithms, known as hyperparameter optimization (HPO). Several techniques are used for

HPO. Grid, random search, and gradient descent are algorithms that automatically perform HPO.

Two Python libraries, Local Interpretable Model-Agnostic Explanations (LIME) and SHapley Additive exPlanations (SHAP) help explain the model and reduce the "black box" aspect of machine learning. In R, the DALEX package offers Accumulated Local Effects (ALE) plots, as well as SHAP and other tools. In the case of SHAP it only applies to ensemble algorithms such as xgboost. These techniques are not without limitations but are a step in the right direction. Figure 4.1 below, displays the most important predictors with xgboost. (111)

Figure 4.1 Feature importance using SHAP

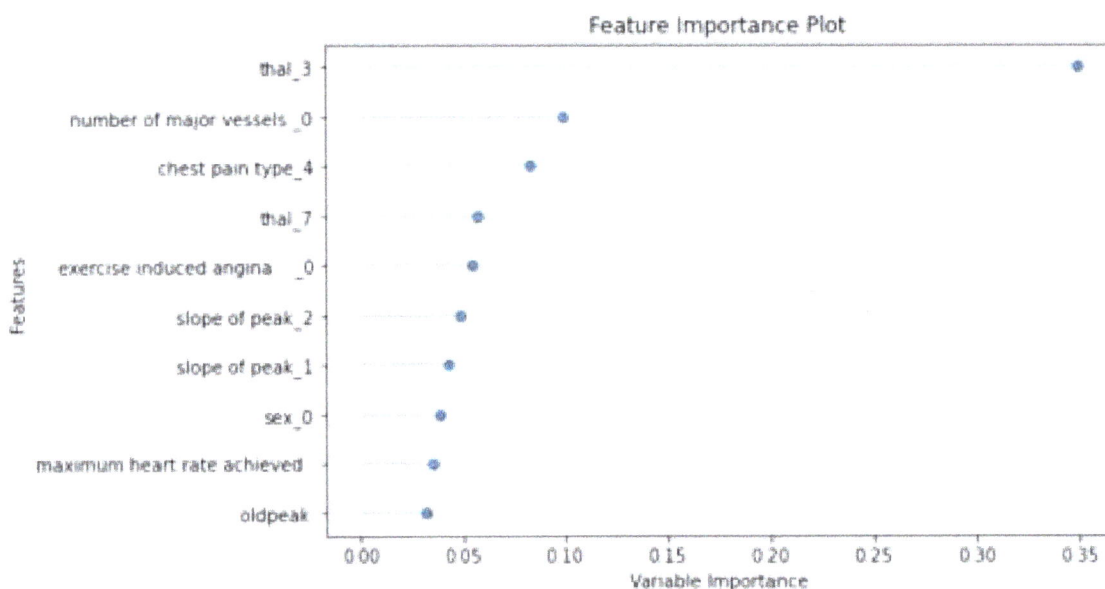

Many of the more accurate model types, such as random forests, gradient boosting models, and neural networks are impossible to interpret directly. Figure 4.2 shows an Accumulated Dependence Profile plot that visualizes how a neural network is using the standardized variable "age" to adjust its prediction as values of age change.

Figure 4.2 Accumulated Dependence Profile Plot showing how the variable Age is used inside a neural network.

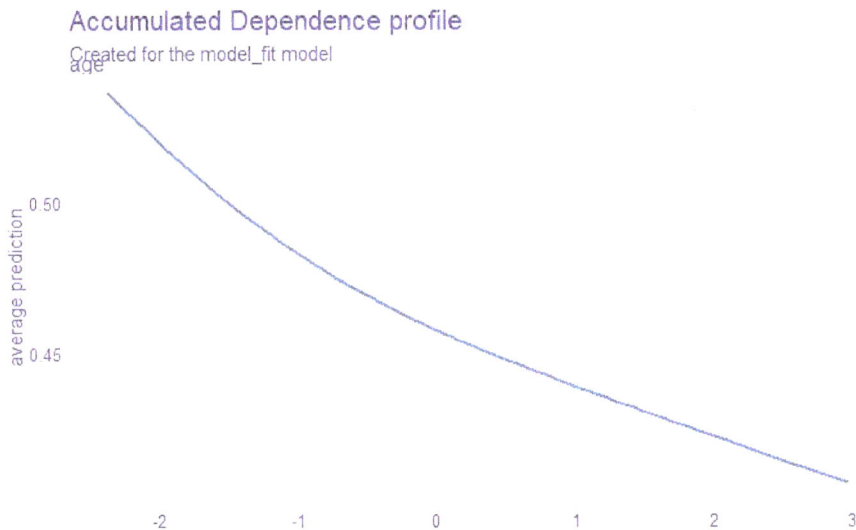

Deploy the Model

First, the model is saved for future deployment. In PyCaret a completed model can be executed locally using the save_model function which saves the transformation pipeline and trained model. R does this using its save function. In BlueSky Statistics, this is accomplished using the Save Model button. Additionally, models can be deployed on cloud platforms such as Google Cloud, Amazon Web Services, and Microsoft Azure. In PyCaret deploying a model in the cloud is as simple as writing `deploy_model`.

Communicate the Results

While tools such as dashboards do help communicate the results of a data science project, the reality is that there needs to be excellent communication and use of human skills, also known as soft skills or eSkills.

SEMI-AUTOMATED DATA PREPARATION AND EXPLORATION SOFTWARE

Example: Trifacta Wrangler

This web-based data preparation platform integrates with Google, Amazon Web Services, Microsoft Azure, Databricks, and Snowflake. Trifacta Wrangler is free and resembles a spreadsheet program with the exception that it analyzes the spreadsheet and makes suggestions. Figure 4.2 displays suggestions related to one liver biomarker ALK_PHOSPHATE where it identified question marks (?) where values should have been and calls those "mismatched." It recommends creating a new column with blank cells replacing the question marks. The process of wrangling requires data cleaning steps that are semi-automated and include joins, creating new columns, formulas, pivots, etc. The steps are part of what is called the Recipe. When wrangling and the Recipe are complete you execute the transformation as a Job to generate the final results. VIDEO (112)

Figure 4.2 Suggestions made by Trifacta

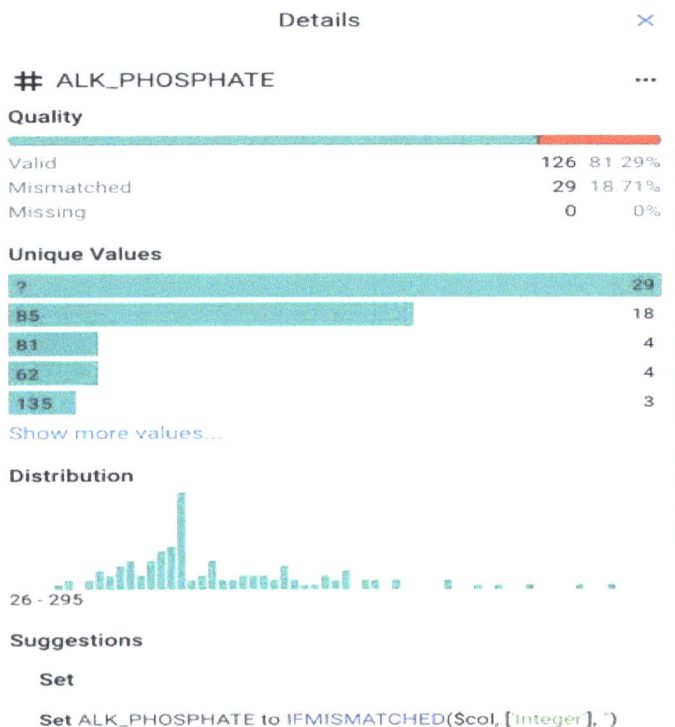

Details   ✕

 # ALK_PHOSPHATE   •••

Quality

Valid	126	81.29%
Mismatched	29	18.71%
Missing	0	0%

Unique Values

?	29
85	18
81	4
62	4
135	3

Show more values...

Distribution

26 - 295

Suggestions

Set

Set ALK_PHOSPHATE to IFMISMATCHED($col, ['Integer'], ')

AUTOML IN PROGRAMMING LANGUAGES

A variety of R and Python packages expedite and automate data preparation and exploration. Most do not have the goal of automating every step in the data science process but these have evolved over time. The following are a sampling of packages that help automate data science processes

1. R programming
    a. Caret stands for Classification And REgression Training and contains functions to streamline the model training process. The package potentially uses up to 30 R packages to implement 238 model types. However, it does not load them all at

start-up (unlike PyCaret). The processes included are: data splitting, pre-processing, feature selection, model tuning, resampling, and variable importance estimation. (13) VIDEO (22)

b. Tidymodels is a newer program than Caret but functions much the same. The processes include: rsample (types of resampling), recipes (transformations for model data pre-processing), parsnip (interface for model creation) and yardstick (measures model performance). (113)

2. Python -
   a. PyCaret is explained in the example below. (15)
   b. Auto-sklearn is based on the machine learning library scikit-learn. It picks the best classification and regression algorithms based on Bayesian optimization. It does perform data preprocessing and hyperparameter tuning but requires more lines of code than PyCaret. (114)

Example: Pycaret 2.0

Pycaret 1.0 was released in the spring of 2020 and by August, version 2.1 was launched. This Python package includes all of the steps of the data science process from data preparation to model deployment. (115) Notable features include:

- Beginner and intermediate tutorials on the website
- About 50 medical and non-medical datasets included. This simplifies data uploads
- Performs supervised (classification and regression) and unsupervised learning (clustering, association rules, anomaly detection, and NLP)
- Requires very little coding as noted in Figure 4.3. To perform k-10 fold cross-validation on the training data and provide classification performance only requires the code `compare.models()`.
- Preprocessing includes the following:
  - Missing value imputation
  - Data type changed as needed
  - One hot, ordinal, and cardinal encoding
  - Normalization and transformation
  - Feature interaction, and feature importance
  - Removing collinearity and PCA
- Select a model and multiple performance outcomes on the training data are displayed (AUC, sensitivity, specificity, precision, F score, and model build time).
- Outcomes can be plotted such as ROC curve, precision-recall curve, etc.
- Performance is then run on the test data with the same outcome data reported
- Models can be deployed on Amazon Web Services, Google Cloud and Microsoft Azure

Figure 4.3 below shows the 41 steps in PyCaret that creates automated data preparation and feature engineering with this simple Python script. False means a step in preparation did not take place. This is an example of AutoML that simplifies data preparation and exploration while also simplifying Python. One of the first steps is to identify the data types in the dataset, then create the setup step.

```
from pycaret.classification import *
exp1 = setup(heart, target = 'Disease')
```

The steps are easy to modify. For example, if a variable should be categorical but PyCaret labels it as numerical then the code would be exp1 = setup(heart, target = 'Disease', categorical _features = ['chest_pain']). (116) VIDEO (27)

Figure 4.3 PyCaret data preparation and feature engineering

	Description	Value			Description	Value
0	session_id	6962		22	Ignore Low Variance	False
1	Target Type	Binary		23	Combine Rare Levels	False
2	Label Encoded	None		24	Rare Level Threshold	None
3	Original Data	(270, 14)		25	Numeric Binning	False
4	Missing Values	False		26	Remove Outliers	False
5	Numeric Features	5		27	Outliers Threshold	None
6	Categorical Features	8		28	Remove Multicollinearity	False
7	Ordinal Features	False		29	Multicollinearity Threshold	None
8	High Cardinality Features	False		30	Clustering	False
9	High Cardinality Method	None		31	Clustering Iteration	None
10	Sampled Data	(270, 14)		32	Polynomial Features	False
11	Transformed Train Set	(188, 25)		33	Polynomial Degree	None
12	Transformed Test Set	(82, 25)		34	Trignometry Features	False
13	Numeric Imputer	mean		35	Polynomial Threshold	None
14	Categorical Imputer	constant		36	Group Features	False
15	Normalize	False		37	Feature Selection	False
16	Normalize Method	None		38	Features Selection Threshold	None
17	Transformation	False		39	Feature Interaction	False
18	Transformation Method	None		40	Feature Ratio	False
19	PCA	False		41	Interaction Threshold	None
20	PCA Method	None				
21	PCA Components	None				

AUTOML IN COMMERCIAL SOFTWARE PROGRAMS

There are many examples of commercial AutoML programs so the following are just a sample of what is available: Google Cloud AutoML, TPOT, RapidMiner Studio, Amazon SageMaker, Microsoft Azure, DataRobot, dotData, KNIME (paid), and H2o Driverless AI (117) (118) (119) (120) (121) (122) (123) (124). All the programs have merit but we will focus on only one commercial example of AutoML.

Example: RapidMiner Studio (TurboPrep)

RapidMiner Studio is a hybrid in the sense that all functions can be performed with visual operators that you connect in a pipeline. However, the platform is automated with data preparation, exploration, and visualization with the functionality known as TurboPrep. This feature can perform most data cleansing, exploration, and visualization functions but it also includes "autocleansing" when activated. This provides the following: remove low-quality variables, dummy code categorical variables, replace missing variables, perform principal component analysis (PCA), and normalize data. Figure 4.4 shows the main TurboPrep screen. VIDEO (125)

Figure 4.4 RapidMiner TurboPrep

Heart_Disease_Prediction

Add new data sets on the left. Details for the selected data are shown below. You can change the data with the following actions. ⓘ

✕ TRANSFORM   ⟋ CLEANSE   ▦ GENERATE   Σ PIVOT   ⊃∗ MERGE   MODEL   CHARTS   CREATE PROCESS   HISTORY   •••

Age Number	Sex Number	Chest pain t... Number	BP Number	Cholesterol Number	FBS over 120 Number	EKG results Number	Max HR Number	Exercise ang... Number	ST depression Number
70	1	4	130	322	0	2	109	0	2.400
67	0	3	115	564	0	2	160	0	1.600
57	1	2	124	261	0	0	141	0	0.300
64	1	4	128	263	0	0	105	1	0.200
74	0	2	120	269	0	2	121	1	0.200
65	1	4	120	177	0	0	140	0	0.400
56	1	3	130	256	1	2	142	1	0.600
59	1	4	110	239	0	2	142	1	1.200
60	1	4	140	293	0	2	170	0	1.200
63	0	4	150	407	0	2	154	0	4
59	1	4	135	234	0	0	161	0	0.500
53	1	4	142	226	0	2	111	1	0
44	1	3	140	235	0	2	180	0	0
61	1	1	134	234	0	0	145	0	2.600
57	0	4	128	303	0	2	159	0	0
71	0	4	112	149	0	0	125	0	1.600

CONCLUSIONS

It is clear that data preparation and exploration occupies the majority of the time spent by data scientists. Automation has impacted almost every step of the data science process and is most commonly called AutoML. The ultimate goal would be not only a system that takes care of basic data preparation and exploration but one that would alert the user with issues and provide solutions. This does imply that the fields of biostatistics and computer science could come to an agreement over challenging issues, such as unified terminologies and how best to handle missing data, imbalanced datasets, etc.

DATA EXERCISES

1. PyCaret https://pycaret.org
   a. Some knowledge of Python would be helpful but not essential
   b. Install Anaconda which will provide you with Python and its packages plus Jupyter Notebooks. Open a Jupyter notebook and following the instructions in this article to predict diabetes which is a dataset included with PyCaret (126)
   c. Use the PyCaret website for directions/tutorials and documentation
   d. Find the best performing model to predict diabetes
   e. List the AUC, sensitivity, and specificity you found

5

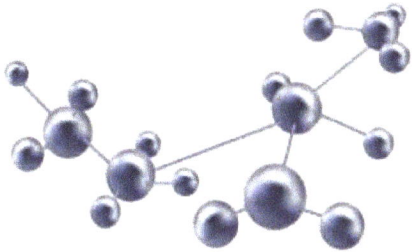

HEALTHCARE DATA RESOURCES

ROBERT HOYT

"Data is a precious thing and will last longer than the systems themselves"
Tim Berners-Lee, inventor of the World Wide Web

This chapter includes the resources found in the Introduction to Biomedical Data Science textbook, plus several additional ones. In this era of "open-data," there are a multitude of available datasets, although they can be limited by privacy (HIPAA) concerns. Most of the federal government datasets are at the hospital, county, or state level, and not at the patient level.

In the master table there are data resources from well-recognized web sites, synthetic patient datasets, and aggregate data from National Health and Nutrition Examination Survey (NHANES). (127) This is one of the few repositories that host patient-level de-identified data. It is strongly recommended that readers adopt as many data preparation and exploration tools as possible. For example, if you plan to use NHANES data you will need tools to upload and analyze SAS transport files (XPT files). Many students/instructors will not have the stats package SAS so downloading is not simple. Fortunately, jamovi will upload these files but you will need to join files together (aggregate) to make sense of the data. NHANES will usually have 9 - 10000 patients for each test performed so it is necessary to have a patient ID so you can combine e.g., demographics with lab tests. There are many options such as writing SQL scripts to combine tables or using a program such as Trifacta Wrangler. The important point is that NHANES data is de-identified patient data covering an incredible breadth of clinical experience, so it should not be overlooked. NHANES has been a research database cited in many published articles.

We encourage readers to explore as many of these resources as possible and to apply some of the tools discussed in this textbook. There is no substitute for getting one's "hands dirty" with data preparation and exploration on multiple different datasets. Government and non-governmental data are listed.

Healthcare datasets	Details
Healthcare Cost and Utilization Project (HCUP) http://www.hcup-us.ahrq.gov	Includes US longitudinal hospital care data with databases, software and online tools
Health Data.Gov http://www.healthdata.gov	Users can search by data category (8) and format(.csv,.xls, zip, PDF, rdf, JSON, html, txt and API
Centers for Disease Control and Prevention http://www.cdc.gov/nchs/data_access/ftp_data.hm	Includes public use files (PUFs) from surveys from multiple government agencies
Centers for Disease Control and Prevention https://www.cdc.gov/DataStatistics/	Various data reports, charts and downloads related to US Health
Centers for Disease Control and Prevention https://gis.cdc.gov/grasp/diabetes/DiabetesAtlas.html	Tracks the prevalence of diabetes by state. Provides a variety of filters, geo-codes, charts, and tables
Centers for Disease Control and Prevention (CDC) Wonder https://wonder.cdc.gov/Welcome.html	Public health-oriented databases
Data.gov https://www.data.gov/	Government repository of open data. Has almost 200,000 datasets that include medical data available to download in various formats
World Health Organization https://www.who.int/data/gho/data/indicators	A myriad of health indicators with visualizations and downloadable datasets
Expert Health Data Programming http://www.ehdp.com/vitalnet/datasets.htm	Host links to about 45 large datasets
Health Services Research Information Central https://hsric.nlm.nih.gov/hsric_public/display_links/722	Has extensive health datasets, statistics, international data and data tools
Vanderbilt Biostatistics Database http://biostat.mc.vanderbilt.edu/wiki/Main/datasets	Multiple health-related datasets are available to download as Excel, ASCII, R, and S-Plus files. Also includes links to international datasets
MIMIC III Critical Care database https://mimic.physionet.org	Repository of more than 40,000 de-identified critical care patient-level inpatient data

Healthcare datasets	Details
CMS Data Navigator https://dnav.cms.gov/Default.aspx	Expedites the search for Medicare and Medicaid data
Gapminder https://www.gapminder.org	Hosts lots of international datasets in .csv format
County Health Rankings and Roadmap http://www.countyhealthrankings.org/	Ranks multiple health measures for US counties. Able to compare counties and download raw data. Data is from 2015-2017 time period
Medicare Data https://data.medicare.gov	Provides downloadable (csv) data to compare hospitals, physicians, nursing homes, hospice, dialysis centers, home health, inpatient rehab, and long term inpatient care. Each category has multiple sub-categories. For example, Hospital Compare has 77 files
National Health and Nutrition Examination Survey (NHANES) https://www.cdc.gov/nchs/nhanes/index.htm	The long-standing project that conducts interviews, physical and lab exams on US citizens. Data is available for download with complete data dictionaries
Harvard Dataset Explorer https://nhanes.hms.harvard.edu/transmart/datasetExplorer/index https://datadryad.org/stash/dataset/doi:10.5061/dryad.d5h62	The Explorer dataset is from 1999-2006 NHANES data that includes 1100 attributes on 41,000+ patients. Has a variety of online tools to analyze this dataset. Unique for including a variety of environmental pollutants and toxins. Data is downloadable from the second URL
Health Information National Trends Survey (HINTS) https://hints.cancer.gov/about-hints/default.aspx .	Part of the National Cancer Institute. Surveys have been conducted since 2003 on cancer and multiple other topics. The data format for SPSS, SAS, and Stata
National Health Interview Survey (NHIS) https://www.cdc.gov/nchs/nhis/index.htm	Another US national health trend survey tool. Includes an interview but no physical exam or lab data.
University of California, Irvine Repository: https://archive.ics.uci.edu/ml/datasets.html	The site includes 325 validated datasets covering many domains, different sizes, and data types, and different analytical methods, such as classification and regression. These datasets are commonly used for machine learning exercises
KDNuggets: www.kdnuggets.com	The site includes 71 datasets available for free download, from various industries.
The Datahub: https://datahub.io/dataset	Managed by the Open Knowledge Foundation, this site hosts more than 10,000 datasets from most industries.

Healthcare datasets	Details
Kaggle: www.kaggle.com	Provides free, interesting datasets for various user interests and analysis.
Data.World https://data.world	New site for creating collaborative data projects with the ability to host data and analyze with embedded SQL. Tools available to link to Tableau, R, and Python languages, and machine learning. Repository for many medical and non-medical datasets
OpenML https://openml.org	Hosts a variety of datasets and ML workflows. Includes the results of multiple ML algorithms run
Sklearn datasets https://scikit-learn.org/stable/datasets/index.html	Python package includes six datasets for analyses
Keras datasets https://keras.io/api/datasets/	Includes seven datasets appropriate for deep learning
Google Dataset Search https://toolbox.google.com/datasetsearch	Google search feature for a variety of datasets, to include health-related. You can search by last updated, format, usage rights and topic. You can also search by task e.g., regression
Google datasets https://ai.google/tools/datasets/	Wide offering generally used to train machine learning and AI
Microsoft Open Datasets https://msropendata.com	Covers categories of computer science, information science, physics, and social science
Open Datasets on GitHub https://github.com/awesomedata/awesome-public-datasets	Extensive list in multiple categories
PyCaret https://pycaret.org	This unique Python package comes with 50 datasets for supervised and unsupervised learning
Synthea https://synthea.mitre.org/downloads	Data on 1,000 synthetic patients can be downloaded that includes conditions, vital signs, medications, encounters, etc. Also, has a 10K COVID-19 dataset
Dataset list https://www.datasetlist.com/	Extensive machine learning datasets that are non-medical
Fast.ai. Datasets https://course.fast.ai/datasets.html	Image, NLP and image localization libraries
NLP datasets https://github.com/niderhoff/nlp-datasets	Primarily raw data for NLP

Healthcare datasets	Details
Kaggle healthcare datasets https://www.kaggle.com/tags/healthcare	Variety of datasets used for Kaggle competitions
SEER datasets https://seer.cancer.gov/explorer/	National Cancer datasets
Oasis imaging datasets http://www.oasis-brains.org/	Open-source neuroimaging data
BigML datasets https://bigml.com/gallery/datasets/healthcare	Healthcare data with spreadsheet-like functionality
Aylward Image Repository http://www.aylward.org/home	Image repository created by Stephen Aylward PhD

APPENDIX: DATA CHECKLIST

DATA PREPARATION & EXPLORATION STEPS	CHECKLIST
DEFINING THE PROBLEM	
Is there a working hypothesis or a well-defined problem?	❏
What type of analysis is needed?	❏
Explorative?	❏
Causative?	❏
Predictive analytics?	❏
Prescriptive analytics?	❏
Is there staff and C-suite buy-in?	❏
Is there a business case for finding a solution to the problem?	❏
Is there a practical and affordable approach?	❏
LOCATING AND RETRIEVING DATA	
Are there data privacy concerns?	❏
What is the data format?	❏
Structured data?	❏
Unstructured data?	❏
Who owns the data?	❏
Did you consider confounding variables?	❏
Does the data require extract, transfer, and load (ETL)?	❏
Does the data require SQL queries?	❏
DATA PREPARATION	
What is the file type?	❏
Will the file type need conversion?	❏
Are the data in a flat file or database?	❏
How many rows and columns are there in this dataset?	❏
What are the data types (numerical, categorical, etc.) in the dataset?	❏
Is there a data dictionary?	❏
Does each column have a header that makes sense with no spaces?	❏
Did you visualize the data with univariate and bivariate plots?	❏
Does the dataset include the units/values of the data?	❏
Is there a target or outcome column?	❏

Descriptive statistics?	❏
Do the minimum and maximum values make sense?	❏
Are the mean and median similar?	❏
How large is each variable's standard deviation?	❏
What is the distribution of the data?	❏
Normally distributed?	❏
Skewed to the right or left?	❏
If skewed, do you need to transform the data?	❏
Are there outliers?	❏
Are there duplicates?	❏
Are the data on different scales?	❏
Does the data require standardization?	❏
Do the data need to be combined by stacking or joining?	❏
Does the data require a pivot table?	❏
Did you clean up incorrect cell data?	❏
Did you prevent data leakage?	❏
How did you handle missing data?	❏
DATA EXPLORATION	
Do you have high correlations between predictors?	❏
Do you have high correlations between the predictors and the outcome?	❏
Do data need to be encoded?	❏
Dummy encoding?	❏
One hot encoding?	❏
Do data need to be placed in bins?	❏
Do you have too many predictors and need dimension reduction?	❏
Do you have a class imbalance problem?	❏

GLOSSARY

Term	Definition	Origin
Algorithm	An algorithm is a set of instructions designed to perform a specific task. This can be a simple process, such as multiplying two numbers, or a complex operation, such as playing a compressed video file.	Tech Terms
ANOVA	Analysis of Variance (ANOVA) is a statistical method used to test differences between two or more means by testing if the variance between the means is significantly greater than the variance within them.	Onlinestatbook
Area under the curve (AUC)	The accuracy of the test depends on how well the test separates the group being tested into those with and without the disease in question. Accuracy is measured by the area under the ROC curve. An area of 1 represents a perfect test; an area of .5 represents a worthless test	University of Nebraska Medical Center
ASCII	ASCII is a character encoding that uses numeric codes to represent characters. These include upper and lowercase English letters, numbers, and punctuation symbols.	Tech Terms
Binning	A way to group numbers of more or less continuous values into a smaller number of "bins". For example, if you have data about a group of people, you might want to arrange their ages into a smaller number of age intervals	Wikipedia
Box plot	A box plot is a graphical rendition of statistical data based on the minimum, first quartile, median, third quartile, and maximum. The term "box plot" comes from the fact that the graph looks like a rectangle with lines extending from the top and bottom. Because of the extending lines, this type of graph is sometimes called a box-and-whisker plot	WhatIs.com
C-suite	C-suite refers to the executive-level managers within a company. Common c-suite executives include chief executive officer (CEO), chief financial officer (CFO), chief operating officer (COO), and chief information officer (CIO)	Investopedia
Categorical data	Categorical variables represent types of data which may be divided into groups. Examples of categorical variables are race, sex, age group, and educational level.	Yale University
Chi-square test	A chi-square test for independence compares two variables in a contingency table to see if they are related. In a more general sense, it tests to see whether distributions of categorical variables differ from each other.	Statistic How To

Term	Definition	Origin
Class imbalance	This is a scenario where the number of observations belonging to one class is significantly lower than those belonging to the other classes.	Analytics Vidhya
Classification	Is the problem of identifying to which of a set of categories (sub-populations) a new observation belongs, on the basis of a training set of data containing observations (or instances) whose category membership is known. Examples are assigning a given email to the "spam" or "non-spam" class, and assigning a diagnosis to a given patient based on observed characteristics of the patient (sex, blood pressure, presence or absence of certain symptoms,etc.)	Wikipedia
Comma separated value	Is a type of data format in which each piece of data is separated by a comma. This is a popular format for transferring data from one application to another, because most database systems are able to import and export comma-delimited data.	Webopedia
Data leakage	Data leakage is when information from outside the training dataset is used to create the model.	Machine Learning Mastery
Data normality	In statistics, normality tests are used to determine if a data set is well-modeled by a normal distribution and to compute how likely it is for a random variable underlying the data set to be normally distributed.	Wikipedia
Data science	Data science is the study of data. It involves developing methods of recording, storing, and analyzing data to effectively extract useful information	Tech Terms
Data visualization	Data visualization is the graphical representation of information and data. By using visual elements like charts, graphs, and maps, data visualization tools provide an accessible way to see and understand trends, outliers, and patterns in data.	Tableau
Data wrangling	Data wrangling is the process of cleaning, structuring and enriching raw data into a desired format for better decision making in less time	Trifacta
Density plot	A density plot is a representation of the distribution of a numeric variable. It uses a kernel density estimate to show the probability density function of the variable	Data to Viz
Descriptive statistics	The analysis of data that helps describe, show or summarize data in a meaningful way such that, for example, patterns might emerge from the data. Descriptive statistics do not, however, allow us to make conclusions beyond the data we have analysed or reach conclusions regarding any hypotheses we might have made. They are simply a way to describe our data.	Laerd Statistics

Term	Definition	Origin
Dimension Reduction	A series of techniques in machine learning and statistics to reduce the number of random variables to consider. It involves feature selection and feature extraction.	Techopedia
Encoding	Is the process of converting the data or a given sequence of characters, symbols, alphabets etc., into a specified format, for the secured transmission of data	Tutorials Point
Feature scaling	Changing the scale of the variables, usually to put them all on the same scale which prevents those on large scales becoming overly influential in modeling.	Wikipedia
Generative adversarial networks	Unsupervised learning task in machine learning that involves automatically discovering and learning the regularities or patterns in input data in such a way that the model can be used to generate or output new examples that plausibly could have been drawn from the original dataset.	Machine Learning Mastery
Histogram	Represents the frequency of occurrence of specific phenomena which lie within a specific range of values, which are arranged in consecutive and fixed intervals. The frequency of the data occurrence is represented by a bar, hence it looks very much like a bar graph.	Techopedia
Imputation	Is replacing missing values with the mean or median values of the dataset at large, or some similar summary statistic.	Kaggle
JavaScript Object Notation	JSON, or JavaScript Object Notation, is a minimal, readable format for structuring data. It is used primarily to transmit data between a server and web application, as an alternative to XML	SquareSpace
Kurtosis	The peakedness or flatness of the graph of a frequency distribution especially with respect to the concentration of values near the mean as compared with the normal distribution	Merriam-Webster
LIME	The acronym LIME, which stands for Local Interpretable Model-Agnostic Explanations, is a specific type of algorithm mode or technique that can help to address the black box problem in machine learning.	Techopedia
Machine learning model	Machine learning models are output by algorithms and consist of model data and a prediction algorithm.	Machine Learning Mastery
NHANES	The National Health and Nutrition Examination Survey (NHANES) is a program of studies designed to assess the health and nutritional status of adults and children in the United States	CDC
Normalization	Rescaling data to have values between 0 and 1. This is also called feature scaling. Confusingly, this is also often referred to as normalization. May also refer to making the variable's distribution more normal, perhaps by taking the logarithm.	Statistics How To

Term	Definition	Origin
Numerical data	Continuous data such as height, weight, blood pressure, etc.	Socratic
Outlier	A data point that is distinctly separate from the rest of the data. One definition of outlier is any data point more than 1.5 interquartile ranges (IQRs) below the first quartile or above the third quartile.	Math Words
Pearson correlation	Statistical test that measures the statistical relationship, or association, between two continuous variables.	Statistics Solutions
Pivot tables	Spreadsheet feature that allows data tables to be rearranged in many ways for different views of the same data.	Business Dictionary
Principal Component Analysis	Principal component analysis aims at reducing a large set of variables to a small set that still contains most of the information in the large set. The new variables have zero correlation, which is helpful for models that have trouble dealing with correlated predictors.	NIST
Python language	Is an interpreted, object-oriented programming language similar to PERL, that has gained popularity because of its clear syntax and readability.	WhatIs
R language	A language that focuses on statistical analysis and machine learning. Its dynamic, interpreted status makes it rather slow, but it is usually used to run methods which are implemented in C and FORTRAN, two static, compiled, high speed languages.	R-Project
Regression	Is a set of statistical processes for estimating the relationships between a dependent variable (often called the 'outcome variable') and one or more independent variables (often called 'predictors', 'covariates', or ' features')	Wikipedia
SHAP	SHAP (SHapley Additive exPlanations) is a theoretic approach to explain the output of any machine learning model.	SHAP
Skewness	A measure of asymmetry (or skewness) quantifies asymmetry in a data set (how much the data is "skewed" to one side of the mean).	Universal Class
SMOTE	Synthetic Minority Oversampling Technique. This is a statistical technique for increasing the number of cases in your dataset in a balanced way. The module works by generating new instances from existing minority cases that you supply as input.	Microsoft
Spearman correlation	A measure of the strength of the linear relationship between the ranks of two variables. A value of +1 indicates a perfect positive relationship, -1 a perfect negative one, and 0 no relationship.	Laerd Statistics
Spreadsheet	Is a computer application for organization, analysis and storage of data in tabular form.	Wikipedia
SQL	Structured Query Language is a way to select data and generate reports from a relational database. Its form is SELECT var1 var2 FROM table_name WHERE logical_condition_is_true.	Techopedia

Term	Definition	Origin
Standardization	Transformations which put all variables on a single scale, such as -3 to +3, or 0 to 1.	Machine Learning Mastery
Statistical package	A set of pre-written statistical routines, usually combined with data management and visualization capabilities.	University of South Australia
Summary statistics	Descriptive statistics such as the frequency, percent, and mode in categorical data, and mean, median, mode, standard deviation, and variance in numeric data.	Math is Fun

REFERENCES

1. Hoyt R, Muenchen R. Introduction to Biomedical Data Science. Informatics Education; 2019.

2. Mayo M. The Data Science Process, Rediscovered - KDnuggets [Internet]. KDnuggets. [cited 2020 Jul 19]. Available from: https://www.kdnuggets.com/the-data-science-process-rediscovered.html/

3. Simplilearn. Data Science In 5 Minutes | Data Science For Beginners | What Is Data Science? | Simplilearn [Internet]. Youtube; 2018 [cited 2020 Oct 27]. Available from: https://www.youtube.com/watch?v=X3paOmcrTjQ

4. Gil Press. Cleaning Big Data: Most Time-Consuming, Least Enjoyable Data Science Task, Survey Says. 2016 Mar 23 [cited 2020 Jul 5]; Available from: https://www.forbes.com/sites/gilpress/2016/03/23/data-preparation-most-time-consuming-least-enjoyable-data-science-task-survey-says/

5. David FN, Tukey JW. Exploratory Data Analysis [Internet]. Vol. 33, Biometrics. 1977. p. 768. Available from: http://dx.doi.org/10.2307/2529486

6. OpenRefine [Internet]. [cited 2020 Jul 5]. Available from: https://openrefine.org/

7. Wikimedian in Residence University of Edinburgh. OpenRefine Beginners Tutorial [Internet]. Youtube; 2019 [cited 2020 Oct 27]. Available from: https://www.youtube.com/watch?v=wfS1qTKFQol

8. Data Wrangling | Prepare Raw & Diverse Data Faster [Internet]. Trifacta. [cited 2020 Jul 5]. Available from: https://www.trifacta.com/

9. Trifacta. Getting Started with Trifacta Wrangler [Internet]. Youtube; 2018 [cited 2020 Oct 27]. Available from: https://www.youtube.com/watch?v=Y72qtcCxDb0

10. Microsoft Excel, Spreadsheet Software, Excel Free Trial [Internet]. [cited 2020 Jul 5]. Available from: https://www.microsoft.com/en-us/microsoft-365/excel

11. Google Sheets: Free Online Spreadsheets for Personal Use [Internet]. [cited 2020 Aug 6]. Available from: https://www.google.com/sheets/about/

12. FrontlineSolvers. Overview of XLMiner Platform Add-in for Excel [Internet]. Youtube; 2015 [cited 2020 Oct 27]. Available from: https://www.youtube.com/watch?v=ehe2RYnBcXs

13. jamovi - Stats. Open. Now [Internet]. [cited 2020 Aug 6]. Available from: https://www.jamovi.org/

14. Home [Internet]. [cited 2020 Aug 6]. Available from: https://www.blueskystatistics.com/

15. Andy Luttrell. PSYS 241: JAMOVI Tutorial 2 - Data and Descriptives [Internet]. Youtube; 2018 [cited 2020 Oct 27]. Available from: https://www.youtube.com/watch?v=3amJB6YuSOI

16. freeCodeCamp.org. jamovi for Data Analysis - Full Tutorial [Internet]. Youtube; 2019 [cited 2020 Oct 27]. Available from: https://www.youtube.com/watch?v=mZomeS0tLxY

17. jamovi > datalab.cc [Internet]. [cited 2020 Oct 27]. Available from: https://datalab.cc/jamovi/

18. Smart Vision Europe. Introduction to BlueSky Statistics [Internet]. Youtube; 2016 [cited 2020 Oct 27]. Available from: https://www.youtube.com/watch?v=6hOXuvBh178

19. What is R? [Internet]. [cited 2020 Aug 6]. Available from: https://www.r-project.org/about.html

20. Welcome to Python.org [Internet]. [cited 2020 Aug 6]. Available from: https://www.python.org/

21. Kuhn M. The caret Package [Internet]. 2019 [cited 2020 Jul 5]. Available from: http://topepo.github.io/caret/index.html

22. Open Education Lab. Practical Machine Learning - Caret Package [Internet]. Youtube; 2017 [cited 2020 Oct 27]. Available from: https://www.youtube.com/watch?v=PhjB5c2P_U0

23. A Grammar of Data Manipulation [Internet]. [cited 2020 Jul 5]. Available from: https://dplyr.tidyverse.org/

24. Data School. Hands-on dplyr tutorial for faster data manipulation in R [Internet]. Youtube; 2014 [cited 2020 Oct 27]. Available from: https://www.youtube.com/watch?v=jWjqLW-u3hc

25. Firke S. Simple Tools for Examining and Cleaning Dirty Data [R package janitor version 2.0.1]. [cited 2020 Jul 5]; Available from: https://CRAN.R-project.org/package=janitor

26. Home - PyCaret [Internet]. PyCaret. [cited 2020 Jul 5]. Available from: https://pycaret.org/

27. Data Professor. Quick tour of PyCaret (a low-code machine learning library in Python) [Internet]. Youtube; 2020 [cited 2020 Oct 27]. Available from: https://www.youtube.com/watch?v=4Rn4YMLUjGc

28. pandas - Python Data Analysis Library [Internet]. [cited 2020 Jul 5]. Available from: https://pandas.pydata.org/

29. Joe James. Python: Pandas Tutorial | Intro to DataFrames [Internet]. Youtube; 2018 [cited 2020 Oct 27]. Available from: https://www.youtube.com/watch?v=e60ItwlZTKM

30. Lafuente AS. Exploratory Data Analysis with Pandas Profiling - Towards Data Science. 2020 Feb 9 [cited 2020 Jul 5]; Available from: https://towardsdatascience.com/exploratory-data-analysis-with-pandas-profiling-de3aae2dd ff3

31. Data Professor. Pandas Profiling for Data Science (Quick and Easy Exploratory Data

Analysis) [Internet]. Youtube; 2020 [cited 2020 Oct 27]. Available from: https://www.youtube.com/watch?v=Ef169VELt5o

32. Zerbe RO, Medema SG. Ronald Coase, the British Tradition, and the Future of Economic Method. In: Medema SG, editor. Coasean Economics Law and Economics and the New Institutional Economics. Dordrecht: Springer Netherlands; 1998. p. 209–38.

33. What is ETL - Extract, Transform, Load? Webopedia Definition [Internet]. [cited 2020 Jul 19]. Available from: https://www.webopedia.com/TERM/E/ETL.html

34. Technology for Teachers and Students. Intermediate Excel Skills, Tips, and Tricks Tutorial [Internet]. Youtube; 2017 [cited 2020 Oct 27]. Available from: https://www.youtube.com/watch?v=lxq_46nY43g

35. Prolific Oaktree. Google Sheets - Full Tutorial [Internet]. Youtube; 2018 [cited 2020 Oct 27]. Available from: https://www.youtube.com/watch?v=zs3ku4uVoho

36. jamovi - Stats. Open. Now [Internet]. [cited 2020 Oct 27]. Available from: https://www.jamovi.org/

37. user guide - jamovi [Internet]. [cited 2020 Oct 27]. Available from: https://www.jamovi.org/user-manual.html

38. datalabcc. Descriptive statistics — jamovi [Internet]. Youtube; 2018 [cited 2020 Oct 27]. Available from: https://www.youtube.com/watch?v=srqNCux0ijY

39. Home [Internet]. [cited 2020 Oct 27]. Available from: https://www.blueskystatistics.com/

40. Videos [Internet]. [cited 2020 Oct 27]. Available from: https://www.blueskystatistics.com/category-s/109.htm

41. OpenRefine [Internet]. [cited 2020 Oct 27]. Available from: https://openrefine.org/

42. Heinsman M. Start Wrangling [Internet]. 2018 [cited 2020 Oct 27]. Available from: https://www.trifacta.com/start-wrangling/

43. CRAN - Mirrors [Internet]. [cited 2020 Oct 27]. Available from: https://cran.r-project.org/mirrors.html

44. How To R. Getting started with R and RStudio [Internet]. Youtube; 2013 [cited 2020 Oct 27]. Available from: https://www.youtube.com/watch?v=lVKMsaWju8w

45. :: Anaconda Cloud [Internet]. [cited 2020 Oct 27]. Available from: https://anaconda.org/

46. Simplilearn. Jupyter Notebook Tutorial | Introduction To Jupyter Notebook | Python Jupyter Notebook | Simplilearn [Internet]. Youtube; 2019 [cited 2020 Oct 27]. Available from: https://www.youtube.com/watch?v=3C9E2yPBw7s

47. Asuncion A, Newman D. UCI machine learning repository [Internet]. 2007. Available from: https://archive.ics.uci.edu/ml/index.php

48. JSON [Internet]. [cited 2020 Jul 12]. Available from: https://www.json.org/json-en.html

49. NHANES Questionnaires, Datasets, and Related Documentation [Internet]. [cited 2020 Jul 9]. Available from: https://wwwn.cdc.gov/nchs/nhanes/

50. Extract data from any websites into a spreadsheet [Internet]. Data Miner. [cited 2020 Jul 5]. Available from: https://data-miner.io/

51. Wieringa J. Intro to Beautiful Soup [Internet]. The Programming Historian. 2012. Available from: http://dx.doi.org/10.46430/phen0008

52. HTML ASCII Reference [Internet]. [cited 2020 Jul 5]. Available from: https://www.w3schools.com/charsets/ref_html_ascii.asp#:~:text=ASCII%20is%20a%207%2Dbit,Z%2C%20and%20some%20special%20characters.

53. Contributors to Wikimedia projects. UTF-8. 2001 Nov 22 [cited 2020 Jul 5]; Available from: https://en.wikipedia.org/wiki/UTF-8

54. Convert ASCII to UTF8 - Online UTF8 Tools [Internet]. [cited 2020 Jul 5]. Available from: https://onlineutf8tools.com/convert-ascii-to-utf8

55. data.world [Internet]. [cited 2020 Sep 3]. Available from: https://data.world/datasets/open-data

56. Rawat S. Heart Disease Prediction - Towards Data Science. 2019 Aug 10 [cited 2020 Jul 5]; Available from: https://towardsdatascience.com/heart-disease-prediction-73468d630cfc

57. Kevin Stratvert. Pivot Table Excel Tutorial [Internet]. Youtube; 2019 [cited 2020 Oct 27]. Available from: https://www.youtube.com/watch?v=m0wl61ahfLc

58. Prolific Oaktree. Google Sheets Pivot Tables - Basic Tutorial [Internet]. Youtube; 2018 [cited 2020 Oct 27]. Available from: https://www.youtube.com/watch?v=Tty0RyD1KLw

59. Matt Macarty. Descriptive Statistics in Excel with Data Analysis Toolpak [Internet]. Youtube; 2015 [cited 2020 Oct 27]. Available from: https://www.youtube.com/watch?v=h-RzBhBzJOQ

60. Jalayer Academy. Google Sheets - Basic Descriptive Statistics (Mean, Variance, Standard Devation, etc.) [Internet]. Youtube; 2015 [cited 2020 Oct 27]. Available from: https://www.youtube.com/watch?v=xLQgIYe5Dss

61. Justin Murphy. Intro to R Studio and Basic Descriptive Statistics [Internet]. Youtube; 2012 [cited 2020 Oct 27]. Available from: https://www.youtube.com/watch?v=uwlwNRbaKMI

62. Ryan Noonan. Python Descriptive Statistics & Five Number Summary [Internet]. Youtube; 2019 [cited 2020 Oct 27]. Available from: https://www.youtube.com/watch?v=sZaTLrxBnU0

63. datalabcc. Histograms — jamovi [Internet]. Youtube; 2018 [cited 2020 Oct 27]. Available from: https://www.youtube.com/watch?v=10oomNrNe6w

64. datalabcc. Bar plots — jamovi [Internet]. Youtube; 2018 [cited 2020 Oct 27]. Available from:

https://www.youtube.com/watch?v=SGtGAISq4kA

65. Scott Stevens. Creating a Histogram with Excel - Using the Analysis ToolPak [Internet]. Youtube; 2014 [cited 2020 Oct 27]. Available from: https://www.youtube.com/watch?v=dMYMUR6rIa4

66. Dr. Bharatendra Rai. Data Visualization in R Part-1 [Internet]. Youtube; 2015 [cited 2020 Oct 27]. Available from: https://www.youtube.com/watch?v=EOhAKMwburY&list=PL34t5iLfZddskPZVTm03hed8K9 3RsyP24&index=2

67. CS Dojo. Intro to Data Analysis / Visualization with Python, Matplotlib and Pandas | Matplotlib Tutorial [Internet]. Youtube; 2018 [cited 2020 Oct 27]. Available from: https://www.youtube.com/watch?v=a9UrKTVEeZA

68. Koehrsen W. Visualizing Data with Pairs Plots in Python - Towards Data Science. 2018 Apr 6 [cited 2020 Jul 8]; Available from: https://towardsdatascience.com/visualizing-data-with-pair-plots-in-python-f228cf529166

69. Data Talks. Pairplot - Seaborn [Internet]. Youtube; 2017 [cited 2020 Oct 27]. Available from: https://www.youtube.com/watch?v=cpZExlOKFH4

70. UTSSC. Creating Scatterplots in RStudio [Internet]. Youtube; 2014 [cited 2020 Oct 27]. Available from: https://www.youtube.com/watch?v=yyXtiGCDOBo

71. Computergaga. Create a Heat Map using Conditional Formatting in Excel [Internet]. Youtube; 2017 [cited 2020 Oct 27]. Available from: https://www.youtube.com/watch?v=kkHEdUI7cfQ

72. Brian Henry. Correlation Matrix [Internet]. Youtube; 2016 [cited 2020 Oct 27]. Available from: https://www.youtube.com/watch?v=uc55cnr8A14

73. Ryan Noonan. Python Correlation Heatmaps with Seaborn & Matplotlib [Internet]. Youtube; 2019 [cited 2020 Oct 27]. Available from: https://www.youtube.com/watch?v=UgtjatBt3vY

74. Contributors to Wikimedia projects. NaN. 2002 Apr 15 [cited 2020 Jul 6]; Available from: https://en.wikipedia.org/wiki/NaN

75. Excel VALUE Function [Internet]. [cited 2020 Jul 10]. Available from: https://exceljet.net/excel-functions/excel-value-function

76. Data Preparation for Machine Learning - Machine Learning Mastery [Internet]. Machine Learning Mastery. [cited 2020 Jul 17]. Available from: https://machinelearningmastery.com/data-preparation-for-machine-learning/

77. Moons KGM, de Groot JAH, Bouwmeester W, Vergouwe Y, Mallett S, Altman DG, et al. Critical Appraisal and Data Extraction for Systematic Reviews of Prediction Modelling Studies: The CHARMS Checklist. PLoS Med. 2014 Oct 14;11(10):e1001744.

78. MeasuringU: 7 Ways to Handle Missing Data [Internet]. [cited 2020 Jul 6]. Available from: https://measuringu.com/handle-missing-data/

79. Multivariate Imputation by Chained Equations [R package mice version 3.9.0]. [cited 2020 Jul 6]; Available from: https://CRAN.R-project.org/package=mice

80. DataSets < Main < Vanderbilt Biostatistics Wiki [Internet]. [cited 2020 Jul 6]. Available from: http://biostat.mc.vanderbilt.edu/wiki/Main/DataSets

81. Reddy MA. A Comprehensive guide on handling Missing Values - #ByCodeGarage - Medium. 2019 Jun 6 [cited 2020 Jul 8]; Available from: https://medium.com/bycodegarage/a-comprehensive-guide-on-handling-missing-values-b12 57a4866d1

82. alexisbcook. Handling Missing Values [Internet]. Kaggle; 2020 [cited 2020 Oct 27]. Available from: https://www.kaggle.com/alexisbcook/handling-missing-values

83. Open Data Community [Internet]. [cited 2020 Oct 27]. Available from: https://data.world/community/open-community/

84. Data Science with Tom. What is tidymodels? + how to install | part 1 | tidymodels tutorial intro in R [Internet]. Youtube; 2020 [cited 2020 Oct 27]. Available from: https://www.youtube.com/watch?v=cgjk7w-mPDs

85. Vaughn KM. RapidMiner Go [Internet]. RapidMiner; 2020 [cited 2020 Aug 6]. Available from: https://rapidminer.com/products/go/

86. [No title] [Internet]. Youtube; [cited 2020 Oct 27]. Available from: https://www.youtube.com/watch?v=TGkMTWk1ISA

87. sklearn.feature_selection.SelectKBest — scikit-learn 0.17.1 documentation [Internet]. [cited 2020 Jul 17]. Available from: https://scikit-learn.org/0.17/modules/generated/sklearn.feature_selection.SelectKBest.html

88. sklearn.feature_selection.RFE — scikit-learn 0.23.1 documentation [Internet]. [cited 2020 Jul 17]. Available from: https://scikit-learn.org/stable/modules/generated/sklearn.feature_selection.RFE.html

89. Murray A. How (and Why) to Use the Outliers Function in Excel. 2019 Jan 7 [cited 2020 Jul 8]; Available from: https://www.howtogeek.com/400211/how-and-why-to-use-the-outliers-function-in-excel/

90. Sharma N. Ways to Detect and Remove the Outliers - Towards Data Science. 2018 May 22 [cited 2020 Jul 8]; Available from: https://towardsdatascience.com/ways-to-detect-and-remove-the-outliers-404d16608dba

91. Excel STANDARDIZE Function [Internet]. [cited 2020 Jul 8]. Available from: https://exceljet.net/excel-functions/excel-standardize-function

92. alexisbcook. Scaling and Normalization [Internet]. Kaggle; 2020 [cited 2020 Oct 27]. Available from: https://www.kaggle.com/alexisbcook/scaling-and-normalization

93. Excel LOG Function [Internet]. [cited 2020 Jul 8]. Available from:
https://exceljet.net/excel-functions/excel-log-function

94. sklearn.preprocessing.PowerTransformer — scikit-learn 0.23.1 documentation [Internet].
[cited 2020 Jul 17]. Available from:
https://scikit-learn.org/stable/modules/generated/sklearn.preprocessing.PowerTransformer.
html

95. Radečić D. Top 3 Methods for Handling Skewed Data - Towards Data Science. 2020 Jan 4
[cited 2020 Jul 8]; Available from:
https://towardsdatascience.com/top-3-methods-for-handling-skewed-data-1334e0debf45

96. Yadav D. Categorical encoding using Label-Encoding and One-Hot-Encoder. 2019 Dec 6
[cited 2020 Jul 8]; Available from:
https://towardsdatascience.com/categorical-encoding-using-label-encoding-and-one-hot-en
coder-911ef77fb5bd

97. Dividing a Continuous Variable into Categories [Internet]. [cited 2020 Jul 8]. Available from:
https://web.ma.utexas.edu/users/mks/statmistakes/dividingcontinuousintocategories.html

98. Altman N, Krzywinski M. The curse(s) of dimensionality. Nat Methods. 2018 May
31;15(6):399–400.

99. Steve Brunton. Principal Component Analysis (PCA) [Internet]. Youtube; 2020 [cited 2020
Oct 27]. Available from: https://www.youtube.com/watch?v=fkf4IBRSeEc

100. Imbalanced Classification with Python - Machine Learning Mastery [Internet]. Machine
Learning Mastery. [cited 2020 Jul 7]. Available from:
https://machinelearningmastery.com/imbalanced-classification-with-python/

101. Website [Internet]. [cited 2020 Jul 8]. Available from: https://arxiv.org/pdf/1106.1813.pdf

102. Shad Griffin. A Simple and Easy Guide to Understanding SMOTE [Internet]. Youtube; 2018
[cited 2020 Oct 27]. Available from: https://www.youtube.com/watch?v=W93qhmLjsnA

103. imbalanced-learn [Internet]. PyPI. [cited 2020 Jul 8]. Available from:
https://pypi.org/project/imbalanced-learn/

104. StatQuest with Josh Starmer. Machine Learning Fundamentals: Cross Validation [Internet].
Youtube; 2018 [cited 2020 Oct 27]. Available from:
https://www.youtube.com/watch?v=fSytzGwwBVw

105. Howson C, Idoine CJ, Sallam RL. Augmented analytics is the future of data and analytics.
Gartner; 2017.

106. Truong A, Walters A, Goodsitt J, Hines K, Bruss CB, Farivar R. Towards Automated
Machine Learning: Evaluation and Comparison of AutoML Approaches and Tools. In: 2019
IEEE 31st International Conference on Tools with Artificial Intelligence (ICTAI). 2019. p.
1471–9.

107. AI Platform [Internet]. [cited 2020 Aug 26]. Available from:

https://cloud.google.com/ai-platform

108. Towards AI Team. The Fundamentals of Neural Architecture Search (NAS) [Internet]. Towards AI — The Best of Tech, Science, and Engineering; 2020 [cited 2020 Aug 26]. Available from: https://towardsai.net/p/machine-learning/the-fundamentals-of-neural-architecture-search-nas

109. Brockman G, Murati M, Welinder P, OpenAI. OpenAI API [Internet]. OpenAI; 2020 [cited 2020 Aug 26]. Available from: https://openai.com/blog/openai-api/

110. He X, Zhao K, Chu X. AutoML: A Survey of the State-of-the-Art [Internet]. arXiv [cs.LG]. 2019. Available from: http://arxiv.org/abs/1908.00709

111. Dataman, Dataman. Explain Your Model with LIME [Internet]. Analytics Vidhya. 2020 [cited 2020 Aug 30]. Available from: https://medium.com/analytics-vidhya/explain-your-model-with-lime-5a1a5867b423

112. Shoemaker A. Why Trifacta [Internet]. 2015 [cited 2020 Oct 27]. Available from: https://www.trifacta.com/why-trifacta/

113. Views R. A Gentle Introduction to tidymodels [Internet]. 2019 [cited 2020 Aug 28]. Available from: https://rviews.rstudio.com/2019/06/19/a-gentle-intro-to-tidymodels/

114. ODSC-Open Data Science, ODSC-Open Data Science. Using Auto-sklearn for More Efficient Model Training [Internet]. Medium. 2019 [cited 2020 Aug 29]. Available from: https://medium.com/@ODSC/using-auto-sklearn-for-more-efficient-model-training-b27be72ba479

115. Welcome to pycaret's documentation! — pycaret 2.0.0 documentation [Internet]. [cited 2020 Aug 30]. Available from: https://pycaret.readthedocs.io/en/latest/

116. Rohith P. Machine learning made easier with PyCaret - Towards Data Science [Internet]. Towards Data Science. 2020 [cited 2020 Aug 29]. Available from: https://towardsdatascience.com/machine-learning-made-easier-with-pycaret-907e7124efe6

117. Bisong E. Google AutoML: Cloud Vision. In: Bisong E, editor. Building Machine Learning and Deep Learning Models on Google Cloud Platform: A Comprehensive Guide for Beginners. Berkeley, CA: Apress; 2019. p. 581–98.

118. Olson RS. TPOT [Internet]. [cited 2020 Aug 6]. Available from: http://epistasislab.github.io/tpot/

119. RapidMiner [Internet]. [cited 2020 Aug 6]. Available from: https://rapidminer.com/

120. Wikipedia contributors. Amazon SageMaker [Internet]. Wikipedia, The Free Encyclopedia. 2020 [cited 2020 Aug 6]. Available from: https://en.wikipedia.org/w/index.php?title=Amazon_SageMaker&oldid=964945333

121. DataRobot Automated Machine Learning [Internet]. [cited 2020 Aug 6]. Available from: https://www.datarobot.com/

122. dotData Home [Internet]. [cited 2020 Aug 6]. Available from: https://dotdata.com/

123. Ricciardi C, Cantoni V, Improta G, Iuppariello L, Latessa I, Cesarelli M, et al. Application of data mining in a cohort of Italian subjects undergoing myocardial perfusion imaging at an academic medical center. Comput Methods Programs Biomed. 2020 Jun;189:105343.

124. H2O Driverless AI - Open Source Leader in AI and ML [Internet]. [cited 2020 Aug 6]. Available from: https://www.h2o.ai/products/h2o-driverless-ai/

125. Machine Learning and RapidMiner Tutorials [Internet]. [cited 2020 Oct 27]. Available from: https://academy.rapidminer.com/learn/video/turbo-prep-data-cleansing

126. Ali M. Announcing PyCaret 1.0.0 - Towards Data Science [Internet]. Towards Data Science. 2020 [cited 2020 Aug 30]. Available from: https://towardsdatascience.com/announcing-pycaret-an-open-source-low-code-machine-learning-library-in-python-4a1f1aad8d46

127. National Health and Nutrition Examination Survey [Internet]. 2020 [cited 2020 Sep 1]. Available from: https://www.cdc.gov/nchs/nhanes/index.htm

www.ingramcontent.com/pod-product-compliance
Lightning Source LLC
Chambersburg PA
CBHW051658210326
41518CB00025B/2602